CW00486798

Keto D Cookbook

The Ultimate Guide to Healthy Weight Loss, Burn Fat and Boost Your Metabolism with 51 Delicious and Easy Recipes

MICHELLE YOUNG

PUBLISHED BY: Green Book Publishing LTD

58 Warwick Road
London W5 5PX

Copyright © Michelle Young

Green Book Publishing ®

All rights reserved. No part of this guide may be reproduced in any form without permission in writing from the publisher except in the case of brief quotations embodied in critical articles or reviews.

Legal & Disclaimer

The information contained in this book and its contents is not designed to replace or take the place of any form of medical or professional advice; and is not meant to replace the need for independent medical, financial, legal or other professional advice or services, as may be required. The content and information in this book has been provided for educational and entertainment purposes only.

The content and information contained in this book has been compiled from sources deemed reliable, and it is accurate to the best of the Author's knowledge, information and belief. However, the Author cannot guarantee its accuracy and validity and cannot be held liable for any errors and/or omissions. Further, changes are periodically made to this book as and when needed. Where appropriate and/or necessary, you must consult a professional (including but not limited to your doctor, attorney, financial advisor or such other professional advisor) before using any of the suggested remedies, techniques, or information in this book.

Upon using the contents and information contained in this book, you agree to hold harmless the Author from and against any damages, costs, and expenses, including any legal fees potentially resulting from the application of any of the information provided by this book. This disclaimer applies to any loss, damages or injury caused by the use and application, whether directly or indirectly, of any advice or information presented, whether for breach of contract, tort, negligence, personal injury, criminal intent, or under any other cause of action.

You agree to accept all risks of using the information presented inside this book.

You agree that by continuing to read this book, where appropriate and/or necessary, you shall consult a professional (including but not limited to your doctor, attorney, or financial advisor or such other advisor as needed) before using any of the suggested remedies, techniques, or information in this book.

Table of Contents

RECIPES

Breakfasts & Smoothies

Buttery Coconut Flour Waffles

This buttery coconut flour waffle recipe requires simple ingredients you probably already have in your cupboard. They are fluffy, light, and can be eaten for breakfast or topped off with keto whipped cream for a delightful dessert.

Ingredients: 5 waffles

- 5 eggs separate whites from yolks

- 4 tablespoons coconut flour

- 1 teaspoon baking powder

- 4 tablespoons granulated stevia

- 2 teaspoons vanilla extract

- ½ cup butter melted

- 3 tablespoons milk full fat

Directions:

• In a bowl, mix the egg yolks, coconut flour, stevia, and baking powder.

• Add the melted butter slowly to the flour mixture, mix well to ensure smooth consistency

• Add the milk and vanilla to the flour and butter mixture. Be sure to mix well.

• In another bowl, whisk the egg whites until fluffy.

• Gently fold spoons of the whisked egg whites into the flour mixture.

• Pour mixture into waffle maker and cook until golden brown.

Nutritional info per serving: Calories 278, Fat 26g, Net Carbs 5g, Protein 8g

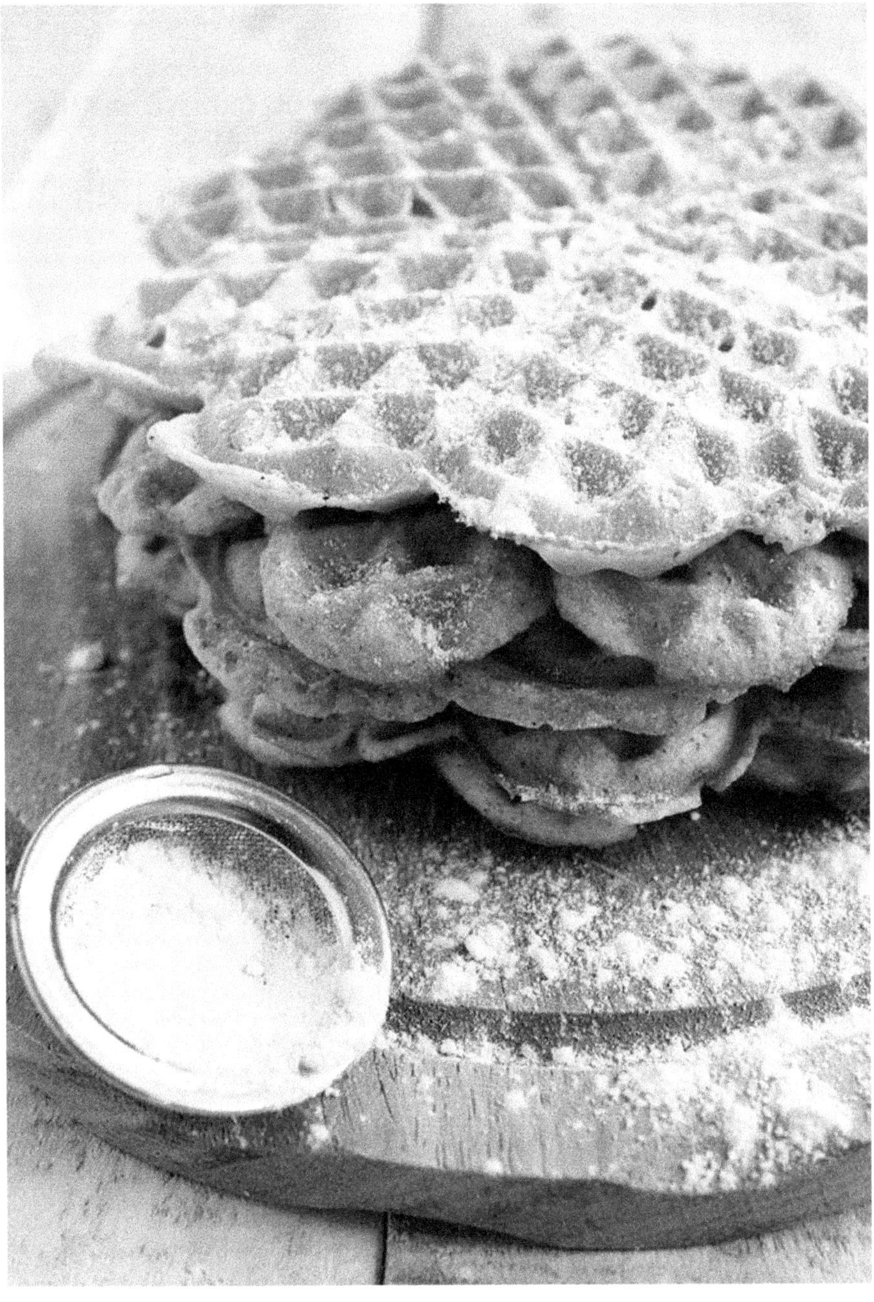

Keto Cheese Omelette

Got cheese, eggs and butter? Then you can whip up delicious in no time! This cheesy keto dish never disappoints. Delight your taste and keep your belly full for hours!

Ingredients: 2 servings

• 3 oz butter

• 6 eggs

• 7 oz shredded cheddar cheese

• Salt and pepper

Directions:

• Whisk the eggs until smooth and slightly frothy. Blend in half of the shredded cheddar cheese. Salt and pepper to taste.

• Melt the butter in a hot frying pan. Pour in the egg mixture and let it set for a few minutes.

• Lower the heat and continue to cook until the egg mixture is almost cooked through. Add the remaining shredded cheddar cheese. Fold and serve immediately.

Nutritional info per serving: Calories 897, Fat 80g, Net Carbs 4g, Protein 40g

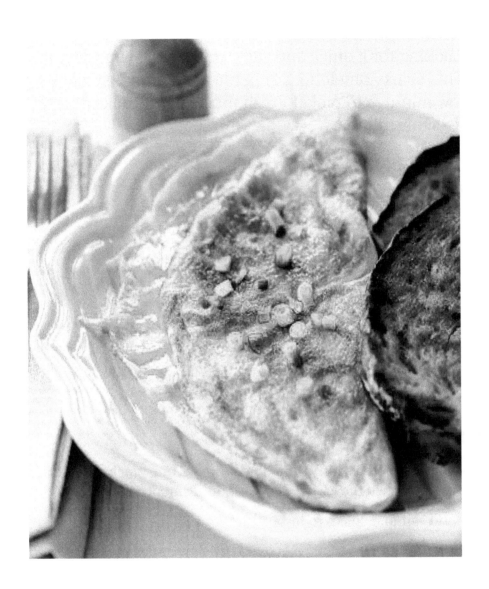

Keto Mushroom Omelette

Looking for a quick and easy way to start your day? This hearty omelette is super healthy, and just takes a few minutes to make! Fresh mushrooms make a delicious filling!

Ingredients: 2 servings

• 6 mushrooms

• 6 eggs

• 2/5 yellow onion

• 2 oz shredded cheese

• 2 oz butter, for frying

• Salt and pepper

Directions:

• Crack the eggs into a mixing bowl with a pinch of salt and pepper. Whisk the eggs with a fork until smooth and frothy.

• Add salt and spices to taste.

• Melt butter in a frying pan. Once the butter has melted, pour in the egg mixture.

• When the omelette begins to cook and get firm, but still has a little raw egg on top, sprinkle cheese, mushrooms and onion on top.

• Using a spatula, carefully ease around the edges of the omelette, and then fold it over in half. When it starts to turn golden brown underneath, remove the pan from the heat and slide the omelette onto a plate.

Nutritional info per serving: Calories 510, Fat 43g, Net Carbs 4g, Protein 25g

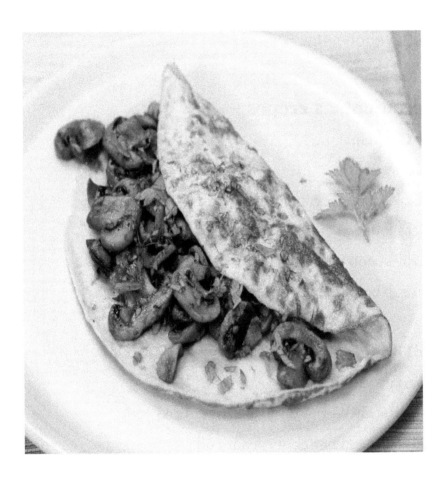

Strawberry Chocolate Keto Crepes

These strawberry chocolate keto crepes are a delectable dessert indulgence. They are made with coconut flour, psyllium husk powder, eggs, sweetener and water, then sprinkled with fresh strawberries and drizzled with melted chocolate.

Ingredients: 2 crepes

For Crepes:

• 3 eggs

• 3 tablespoons coconut flour

• 1 teaspoon sweetener

• 1 tablespoon psyllium husk powder

• 1/3 cup boiling water

For Filling:

• 1 oz dark chocolate

• ½ cup strawberries or raspberries, diced

• ½ tablespoon butter or coconut oil

Directions:

• Mix eggs, coconut flour, sweetener and psyllium husk powder in a bowl. Add in boiling water and mix until well-incorporated.

• In a nonstick pan, add 1 tablespoon oil and turn heat to medium. Once the pan is hot, add in ¼ to ½ of the crepe liquid and allow to cook until the edges begin to brown. Flip over and allow to cook until golden brown. This will take roughly 3-5 minutes per crepe.

• Set cooked crepe aside and repeat until all of the dough is used up.

• If making the strawberry chocolate crepe shown above, melt chocolate in the microwave with butter or coconut oil, in 30 seconds bursts, until fully melted. Be sure to stir between bursts or the chocolate may burn.

• Fill crepes with a handful of berries and a spoonful of chocolate. Fold sides of crepe to close and top with additional berries and chocolate, if desired.

Nutritional info per serving: Calories 167, Fat 12g, Net Carbs 5g, Protein 7g

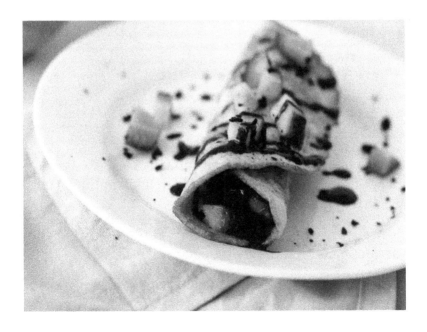

Keto Fried Eggs with Kale and Pork

Eggs and greens, together with the crunch of nuts and crispy pork, deliver with texture and flavor. Make this all-in-one-pan, butter-infused keto wonder any night of the week!

Ingredients: 2 servings

- ½ lb kale
- 4 eggs
- 3 oz butter
- ¼ cup frozen cranberries
- 1 oz pecans or walnuts
- 6 oz smoked pork belly or bacon
- Salt and pepper

Directions:

• Trim and chop the kale into large squares. Melt two thirds of the butter in a frying pan and fry the kale quickly on high heat until slightly browned around the edges.

• Remove the kale from the frying pan and set aside. Sear the pork belly or bacon in the same frying pan until crispy.

• Lower the heat. Return the sautèed kale to the pan and add the cranberries and nuts. Stir until warmed through. Reserve in a bowl.

• Turn up the heat and fry the eggs in the rest of the butter. Salt and pepper to taste. Plate two fried eggs with each portion of greens and serve immediately.

Nutritional info per serving: Calories 1033, Fat 99g, Net Carbs 8g, Protein 26g

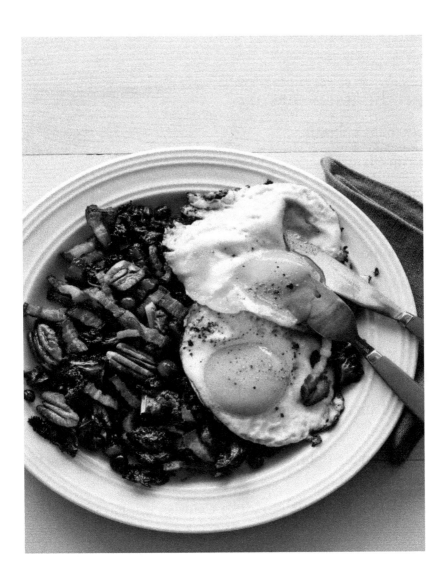

Keto Green Smoothie

A low-carb high fat keto smoothie to have for breakfast or to snack. No sugary fruit, no sweeteners, only low carb veggies, high fat avocado and ginger, lemon and cilantro for that special flavor!

Ingredients: 2 servings

• 1 cup baby spinach

• ½ cup cilantro

• 1 cup cold water

• 1 inch ginger, peeled

• ½ - 1 lemon, peeled

• ¾ English cucumber, peeled

• 1 cup frozen avocado

Directions:

• Add all ingredients to a high speed blender and blend until smooth.

• Store in an air-tight container such as a mason jar in the fridge for up to 3 days.

Nutritional info per serving: Calories 151, Fat 11g, Net Carbs 9g, Protein 3g

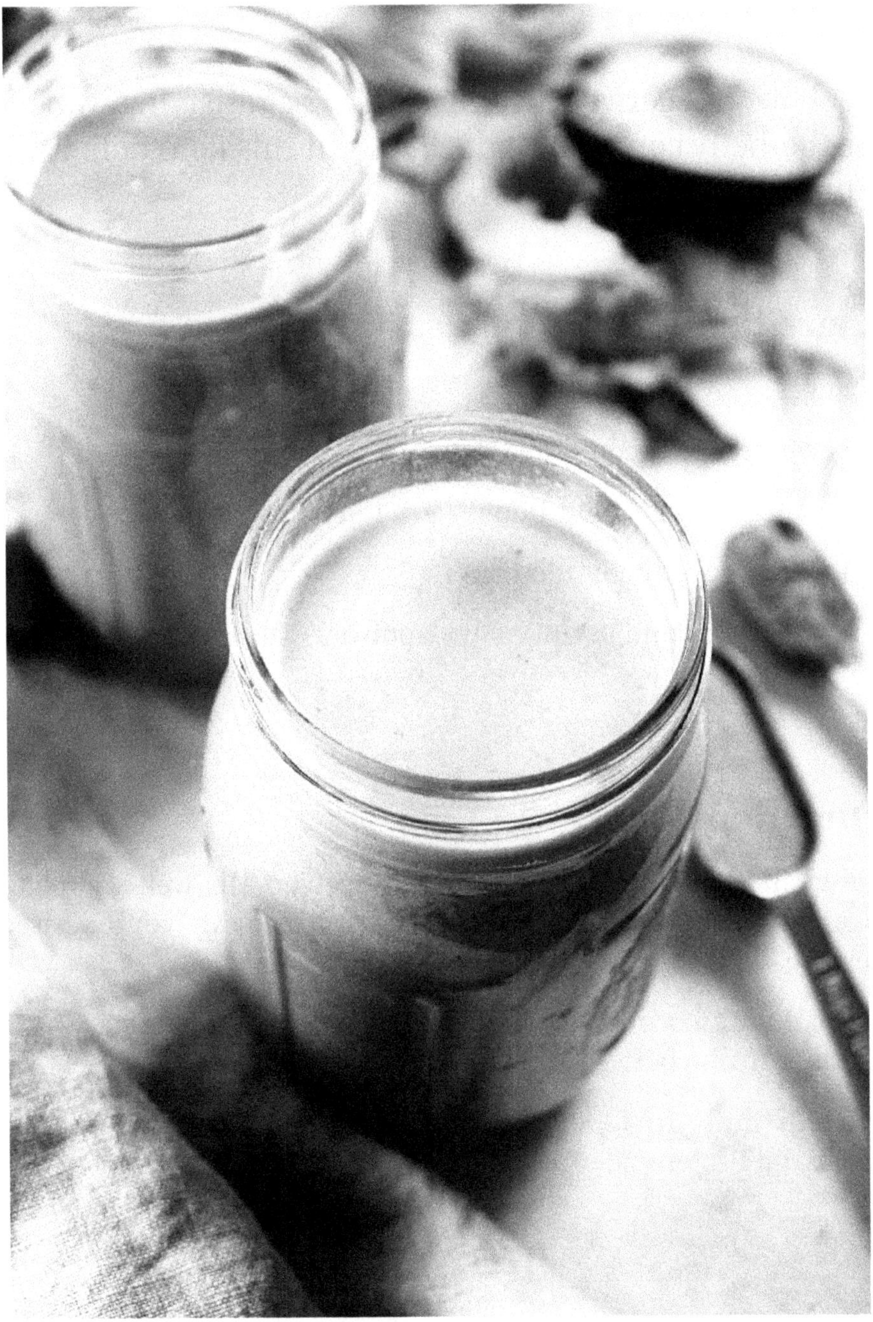

Keto Coconut Porridge

Feel like hot cereal this morning? For satisfying, warm-in-the-belly comfort food, check out this keto delight. Pure happiness in a bowl!

Ingredients: 2 servings

- 2 eggs

- 2 oz butter or coconut oil

- 2 tablespoons coconut flour

- 8 tablespoons coconut cream

- 2 pinches ground psyllium husk powder

- 2 pinches salt

Directions:

• Add all ingredients to a nonstick saucepan. Mix well and place over low heat. Stir constantly until you achieve your desired texture.

• Serve with coconut milk or cream. Top your porridge with a fresh or frozen berries and enjoy.

Nutritional info per serving: Calories 486, Fat 49g, Net Carbs 4g, Protein 9g

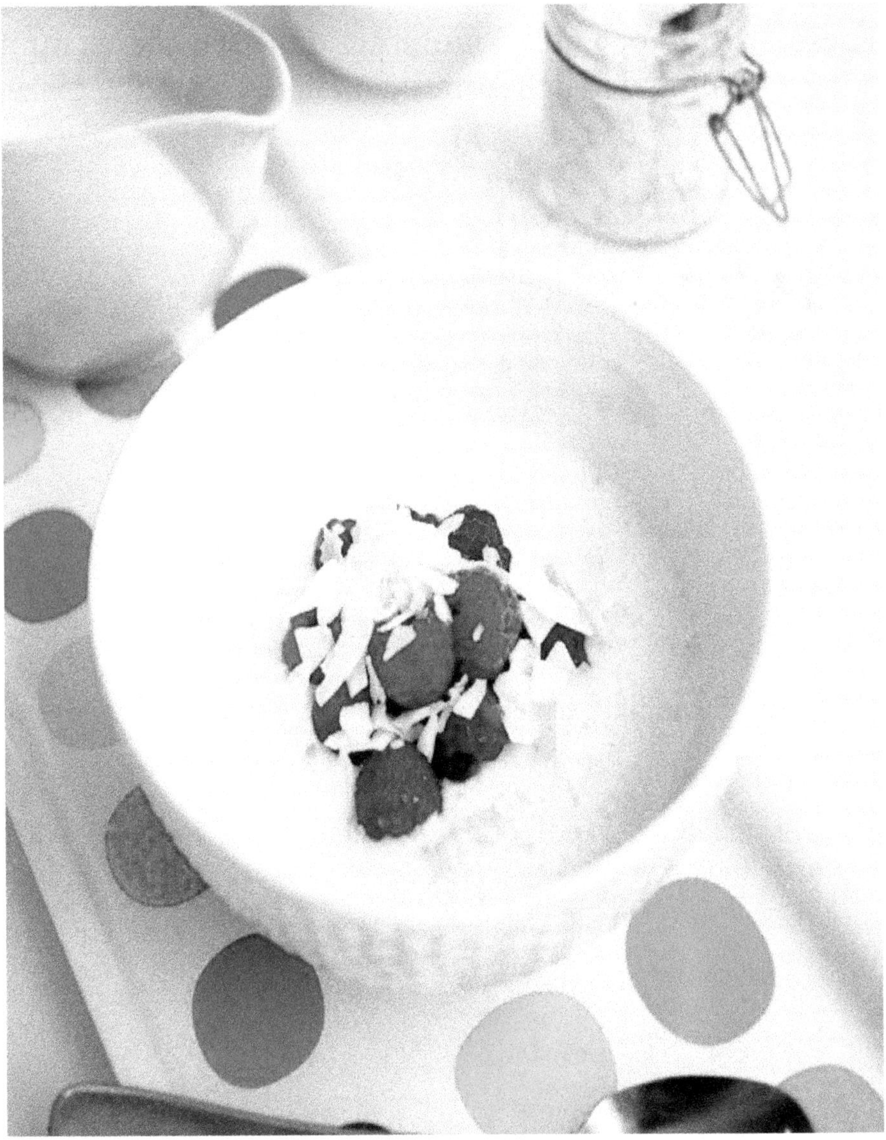

Keto Chocolate Cake Donuts

These keto chocolate donuts are made with coconut flour and dipped in a dreamy sugar-free chocolate glaze.

Ingredients: 8 servings

Donuts:

• 1/3 cup coconut flour

• 3 tablespoons cocoa powder

• 1/3 cup Swerve Sweetener

• 1 teaspoon baking powder

• 4 large eggs

• ¼ teaspoon salt

• ½ teaspoon vanilla extract

• ¼ cup butter melted

• 6 tablespoons brewed coffee or water coffee intensifies the chocolate flavor

Glaze:

• 1 tablespoon cocoa powder

• 1 tablespoon heavy cream

• ¼ cup powdered Swerve Sweetener

• ¼ teaspoon vanilla extract

• 1 ½ - 2 tablespoons water

Directions:

Donuts:

• Preheat the oven to 325 degrees F and grease a donut pan very well.

• In a medium bowl, whisk together the coconut flour, cocoa powder, sweetener, baking powder, and salt. Stir in the eggs, melted butter, and vanilla extract, then stir in the cold coffee or water until well combined.

• Divide the batter among the wells of the donut pan. If you have a six-well donut pan, you may need to work in batches.

• Bake 16 to 20 minutes, until the donuts are set and firm to the touch. Remove and let cool in the pan for 10 minutes, then flip out onto a wire rack to cool completely.

Glaze:

• In a medium shallow bowl, whisk together the powdered sweetener and cocoa powder. Add the heavy cream and vanilla and whisk to combine.

• Add enough water until the glaze thins out and is of a "dippable" consistency, without being too watery.

• Dip the top of each donut into the glaze and let set, about 30 minutes.

Nutritional info per serving: Calories 123, Fat 9.2g, Net Carbs 4.6g, Protein 4.4g

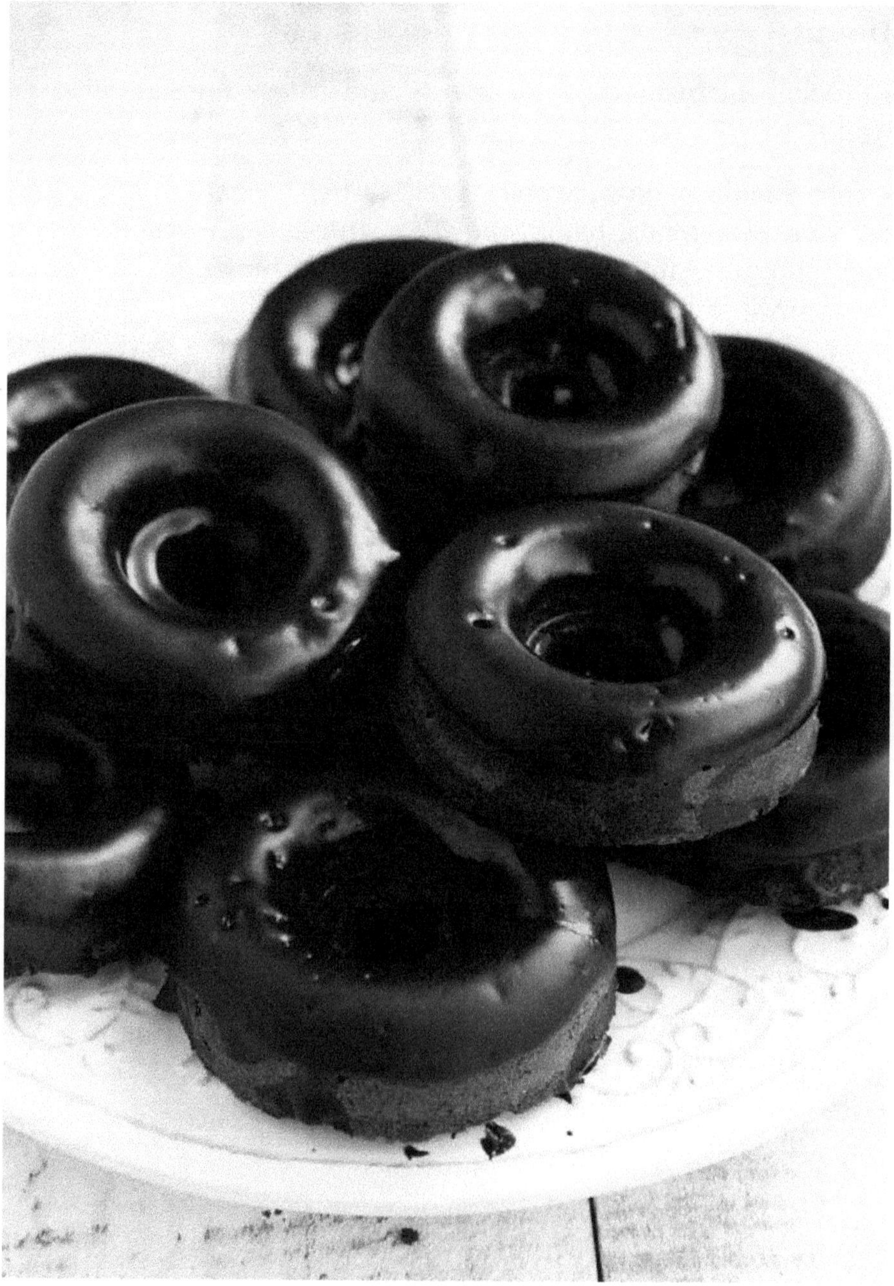

Apps & Snacks

Keto Rosemary Parmesan Crackers

Deliciously low carb, grain-free crackers made with sunflower and chia seeds. This nut-free snack will delight adults and kids alike!

Ingredients: 20 crackers

- ¾ cup Bob's Red Mill raw sunflower seeds
- ¼ cup Bob's Red Mill chia seeds
- 1/3 cup finely grated Parmesan
- 1 tablespoon melted butter
- 1 tablespoon chopped fresh rosemary
- ¼ teaspoon baking powder
- ½ large egg
- ¼ teaspoon garlic powder
- ¼ teaspoon kosher salt

Directions:

- Preheat the oven to 300 degrees F.

- In a high-powered blender or food processor, grind the sunflower seeds and chia seeds until finely ground. Then measure out half cup of the ground sunflower seeds and half cup of the ground chia seeds into a large bowl.

• Stir in Parmesan, fresh rosemary, garlic powder and baking powder.

• Stir in egg and butter until dough comes together.

• Turn dough out onto a large piece of parchment paper and pat into a rough triangle. Top with another large piece of parchment paper. Roll out to about a 1/8 inch thickness, as evenly as you can. Remove top parchment.

• Use a sharp knife or pizza cutter to score into 2 inch squares. Sprinkle with kosher salt. Transfer whole bottom parchment paper to a large baking sheet.

• Bake 40 to 45 minutes, or until edges are golden brown and the crackers are firm to the touch. Remove and let cool completely before breaking apart. They will continue to crisp up as they cool.

Nutritional info per serving: Calories 223, Fat 18.3g, Net Carbs 2.37g, Protein 8.71g

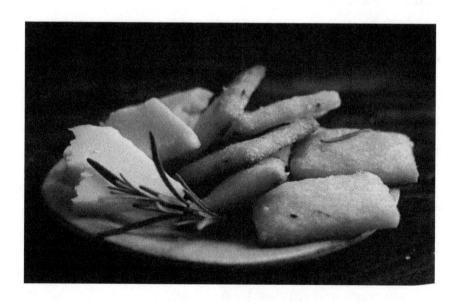

Broccoli Cheddar Bites

Cheesy baked broccoli snacks, great for a brunch, kid-friendly lunch, or party!

Ingredients: 24 bites

- 1 large bunch of broccoli florets
- ½ cup, packed, torn fresh bread
- 2 eggs, lightly beaten
- ¼ cup mayonnaise
- ¼ cup grated onion
- 1 ½ teaspoons lemon zest
- 1 cup, packed, grated sharp cheddar cheese
- ¼ teaspoon freshly ground black pepper
- ½ teaspoon kosher salt

Directions:

• Place 1 inch of water in a pot with a steamer basket. Bring to a boil. Add the broccoli florets. Steam the broccoli florets for 5 minutes, until just tender. Rinse with cold water to stop the cooking. Finely chop the steamed broccoli florets. You should have 2 to 2 ½ cups.

• Place the beaten eggs and the torn bread in a large bowl. Mix until the bread is completely moistened. Add the grated onion, mayonnaise, cheese, lemon zest, salt and pepper. Stir in the minced broccoli.

• Preheat the oven to 350 degrees F. Coat the wells of 2 mini muffin pans with olive oil. Distribute the broccoli mixture in the muffin wells.

• Bake at 350 degrees F for 25 minutes until cooked through and lightly browned on top. If you don't have mini muffin pans, you can cook the bites freeform. Just grease a baking sheet and spoon large dollops of the mixture onto the pan. Baking time is the same.

Nutritional info per serving: Calories 62, Fat 4.8g, Net Carbs 3g, Protein 1g

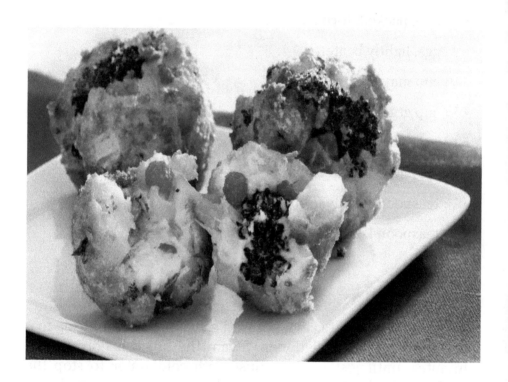

Bacon Wrapped Scallops

Bacon wrapped scallops are elegant enough for a dinner party or a romantic dinner for two and easy enough to prepare on a busy weeknight. In less than 30 minutes you can cook bacon wrapped scallops in the oven to tender, juicy perfection.

Ingredients: 4 servings

• 16 sea scallops

• olive oil for drizzling

• 8 slices bacon, cut in half crosswise

• 8 toothpicks

• Freshly ground black pepper to taste

• Kosher salt to taste

Directions:

• Preheat the oven to 425 degrees F.

• Line a baking sheet with parchment paper. Set aside.

• Pat scallops dry with a paper towel and remove any side muscles. Wrap one scallop in a half slice of bacon and secure with toothpick. Repeat with remaining scallops.

• Drizzle olive oil over each scallop and season with pepper and kosher salt.

• Arrange scallops in a single layer on prepared baking sheet, giving each scallop some room to allow the bacon to crisp.

• Bake 12 to 15 minutes until scallop is tender and opaque and bacon is cooked through. Serve hot.

Nutritional info per serving: Calories 224, Fat 17g, Net Carbs 2g, Protein 12g

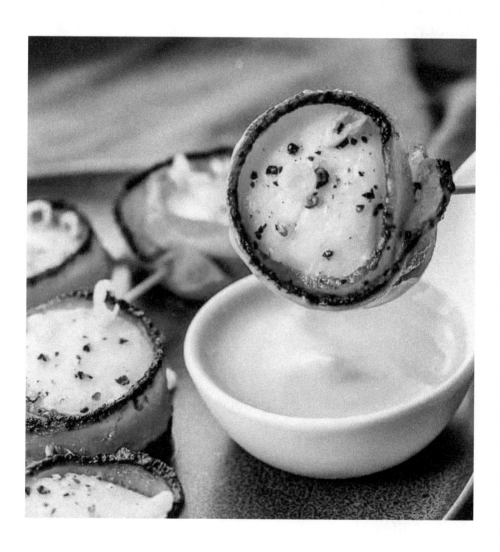

Spicy Deviled Eggs

If you've wondered how to make spicy deviled eggs, this recipe is for you! A spicy sriracha kick and a sprinkle of red chili flakes take creamy deviled eggs from just okay to extraordinary.

Ingredients: 24 egg halves

- 12 large eggs
- 1 tablespoon sriracha sauce
- 1/3 cup mayonnaise
- 1 tablespoon Dijon mustard
- Fine chili flakes
- Fresh chives, minced
- Salt and freshly ground black pepper to taste

Directions:

• Fill a saucepan with enough water to cover eggs by an inch and bring to full boil. Carefully lower eggs into boiling water. Let eggs boil uncovered for about 30 seconds. Reduce heat to low and cover. Simmer for 11 minutes. Transfer boiled eggs to a bowl of ice water. When cool enough to handle, gently break shell apart and peel. If possible, refrigerate eggs overnight, making them easier to cut.

• Once eggs are cool, cut in half lengthwise with a very sharp knife. Carefully spoon yolks out into a small bowl and arrange whites on serving platter.

• In a medium bowl, mash yolks into a paste with the back of a fork. Add mayonnaise, sriracha sauce and mustard; whisk until smooth. Season to taste with salt, freshly ground black pepper and more sriracha if you like.

• Spoon or pipe filling into egg white halves.

• Cover and refrigerate eggs for 2 hours or more (up to 1 day). Once chilled sprinkle generously with fine chili flakes and minced chives. Serve.

Nutritional info per serving: Calories 53, Fat 4g, Net Carbs 0.6g , Protein 2 g

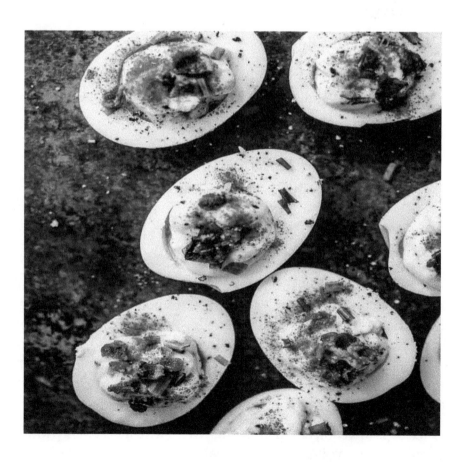

No Bake Low-Carb Zucchini Roll-Ups

Easy no bake low carb zucchini roll ups with guacamole, carrots, celery and mixed greens stuffed in a whole peperoncini! Every bite is so fresh, crunchy and delicious, sometimes you just have to eat on the spot.

Ingredients: 20 roll-ups

- 1 large zucchini

- 1 jar peperoncini

- 1 medium carrot

- Handful mixed greens

- 1 tub guacamole

- 1 single celery stalk

- Fresh dill

Directions:

• Using a peeler slice the zucchini the long way, on all sides to avoid the center. Basically, make 3-4 slices on one side and move on to the opposite side, then the other two sides until you have about 20 slices. Don't discard the middle, just add to your next skillet meal. Set aside.

• Using a mandoline slicer, cut the carrots and celery into thin strips. Set aside.

• Finally, cut the top part off of each peperoncini, make a cut on one side to open and clean seeds out.

Arranging the Roll Ups:

• On a flat surface place one zucchini stip. Spread a dab of guacamole on one end. Place a peperoncini on top of the guacamole, open side up. Fill pocket whole of the peperoncini with guacamole. Add in 1-2 mixed green leaves, 3 strips of carrots, 1-2 strips of celery, fresh dill and roll it tight until you reach the end of the zucchini. If you need help keeping the zucchini roll ups tight in place, add another dab of guacamole on the end part of the zucchini to stick together.

• Do this step until you've used all the ingredients.

• Serve cold and refrigerate leftover for up to 24 hours. The guacamole will darken after this time.

Nutritional info per serving: Calories 234, Fat 4.7g, Net Carbs 4g, Protein 5g

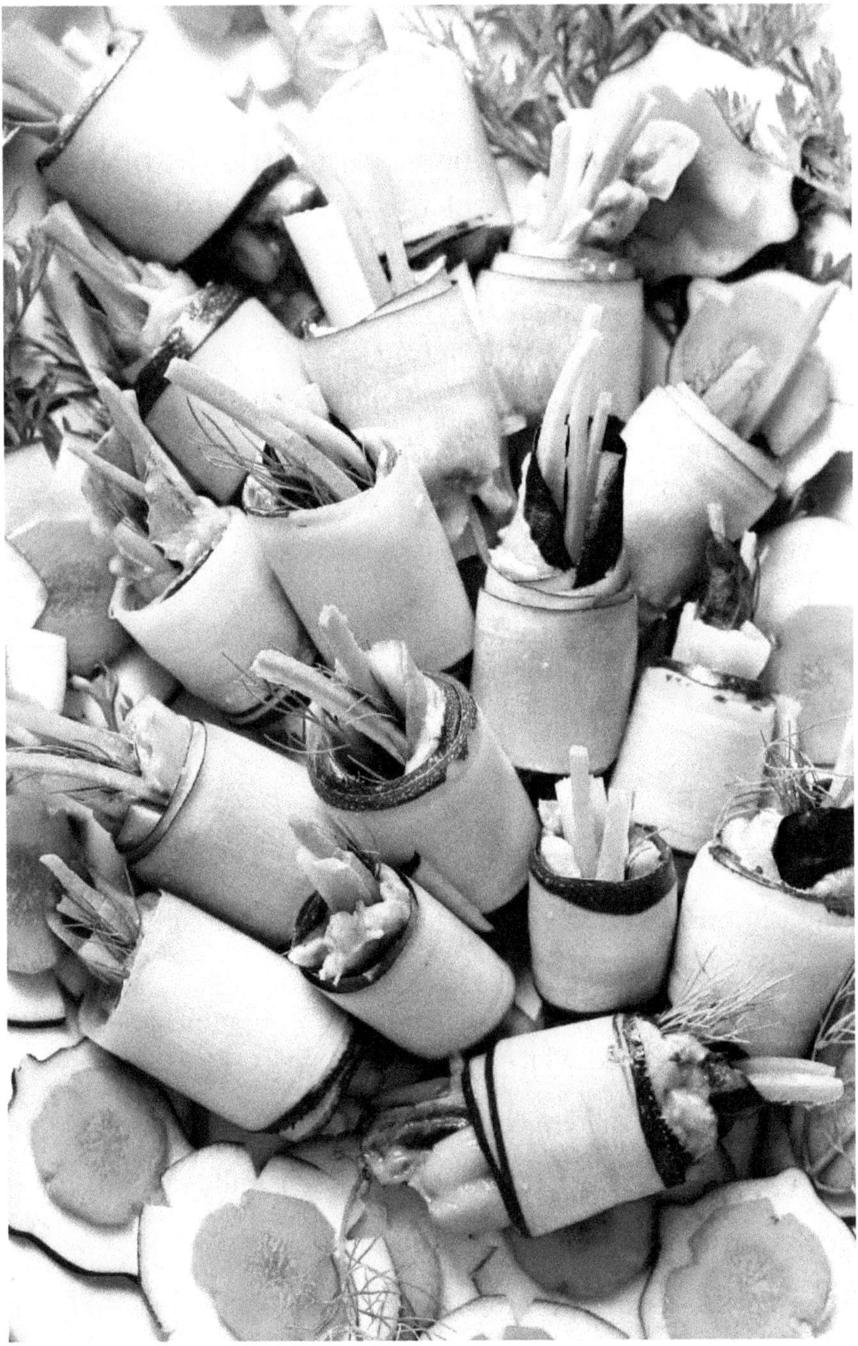

Sweet Pepper Poppers

These sweet pepper poppers are a little bit of heaven! They are low carb, perfect for anyone who is trying to avoid extra carbs.

Ingredients: 6 servings

• 6 large mini sweet peppers, cut in half lengthwise with seeds removed

• ½ cup shredded cheddar cheese

• 3 slices pre-cooked bacon, crumbled

• 1 cup Philadelphia Garden Vegetable Cream Cheese

Directions:

• Preheat the oven to 350 degrees F.

• Slightly oil large baking sheet or cover with a silicone baking sheet/parchment paper.

• Fill each pepper with approximately one tablespoon cream cheese, or until filled. Place on a baking sheet.

• Sprinkle with shredded cheese and bacon.

• Bake for 15 to 20 minutes or until cheese is fully melted.

• Serve warm or refrigerate until serving.

Nutritional info per serving: Calories 65.6, Fat 4.8g, Net Carbs 2.3g, Protein 3.3g

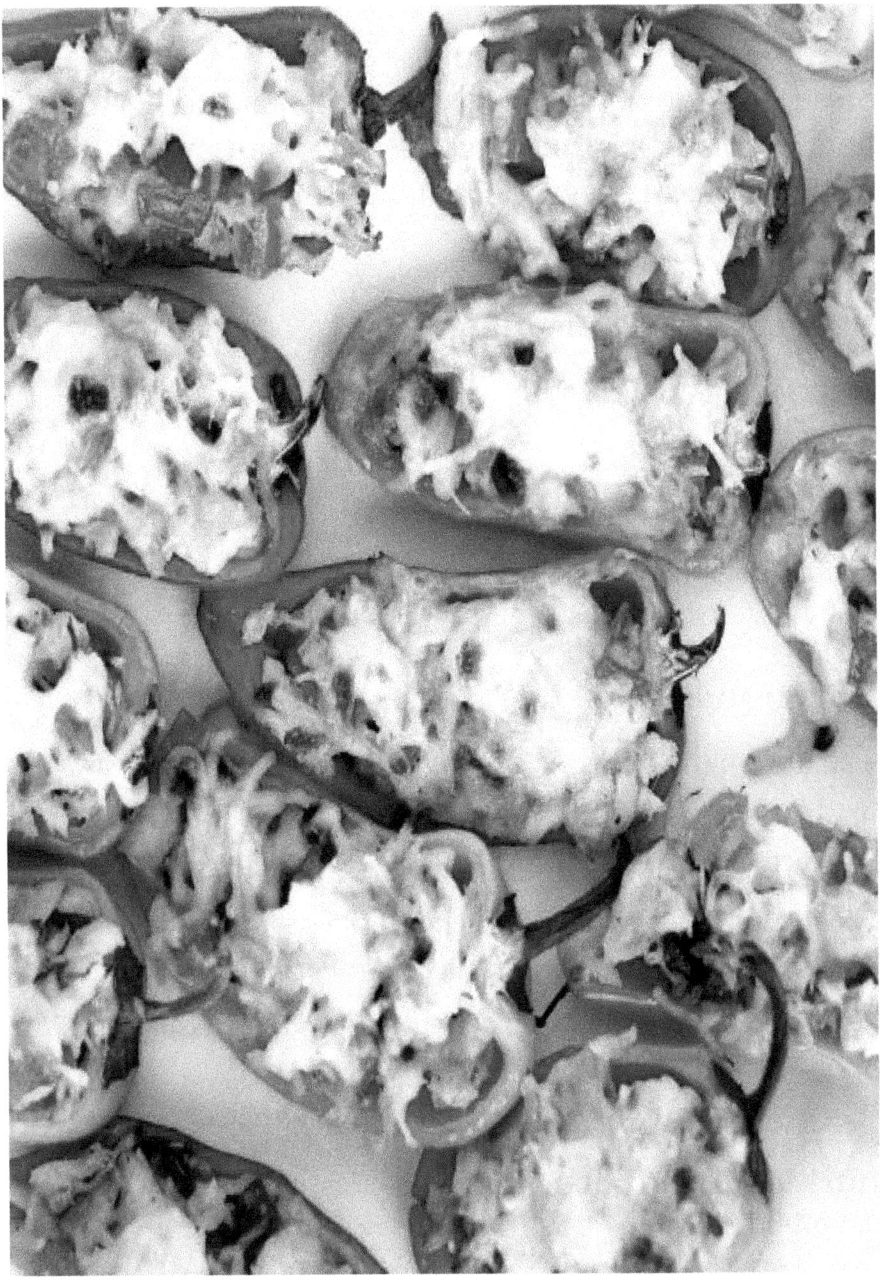

Avocado Deviled Eggs

These avocado deviled eggs are delicious and perfect for the kids. They are full of good fats, from avocado, and protein from the eggs. This makes them a great snack!

Ingredients: 3 servings

• 3 eggs

• 1 avocado

• 1 tablespoon chopped chives

• 1 tablespoon freshly squeezed lime juice

Directions:

• Peel your hard boiled eggs and cut them in half, lengthways.

• Remove the cooked yolk and add to a mixing bowl along with the avocado and lime juice.

• Mash, with a fork, until you achieve the desired texture. Stir in the chopped chives.

• Either spoon the mixture back into the eggs or pipe it into the eggs using a piping bag or zip lock back.

• Serve straight away.

Nutritional info per serving: Calories 156, Fat 3g, Net Carbs 1g, Protein 3g

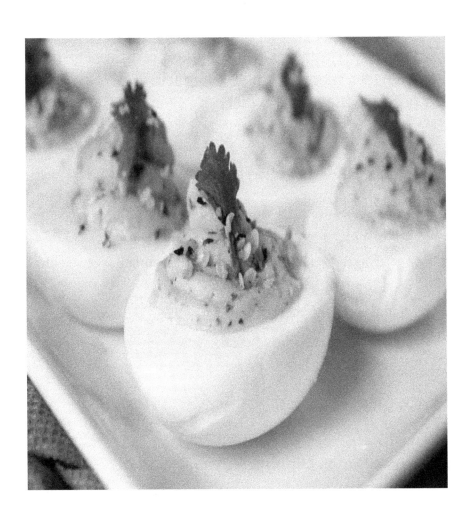

Buffalo Chicken Sausage Balls

These low car, gluten-free Buffalo flavored sausage balls are the perfect recipe for a tasty snack! Make a double batch because they will go fast!

Ingredients: 12 servings

Sausage Balls:

• 2 cups almond flour

• 2 14-oz packages fresh Buffalo-Style chicken sausage, casings removed

• ½ cup crumbled bleu cheese

• 1 ½ cups shredded cheddar cheese

• ½ teaspoon pepper

• 1 teaspoon salt

Bleu Cheese Ranch Dipping Sauce:

• 1/3 cup unsweetened almond milk

• 1/3 cup mayonnaise

• 1 teaspoon dried dill

• 2 cloves garlic, minced

• ¼ cup crumbled bleu cheese

• ½ teaspoon dried parsley

• ½ teaspoon pepper

• ½ teaspoon salt

Directions:

Sausage Balls:

• Preheat the oven to 350 degrees F and line two large baking sheets with parchment paper or tin foil.

• In a large bowl, combine sausage, almond flour, bleu cheese, cheddar cheese, salt and pepper. Mix thoroughly until well combined.

• Roll into 1-inch balls and place about an inch apart on prepared baking sheets. Bake 25 minutes, until golden brown. Serve warm with dipping sauce.

Dipping Sauce:

• While sausage balls are baking, combine mayonnaise, almond milk, garlic, parsley, dill, salt, and pepper in a medium bowl. Stir well and then mix in crumbled bleu cheese.

Nutritional info per serving (4 meatballs per serving): Calories 325 , Fat 25g, Net Carbs 4.3g, protein 20.3g

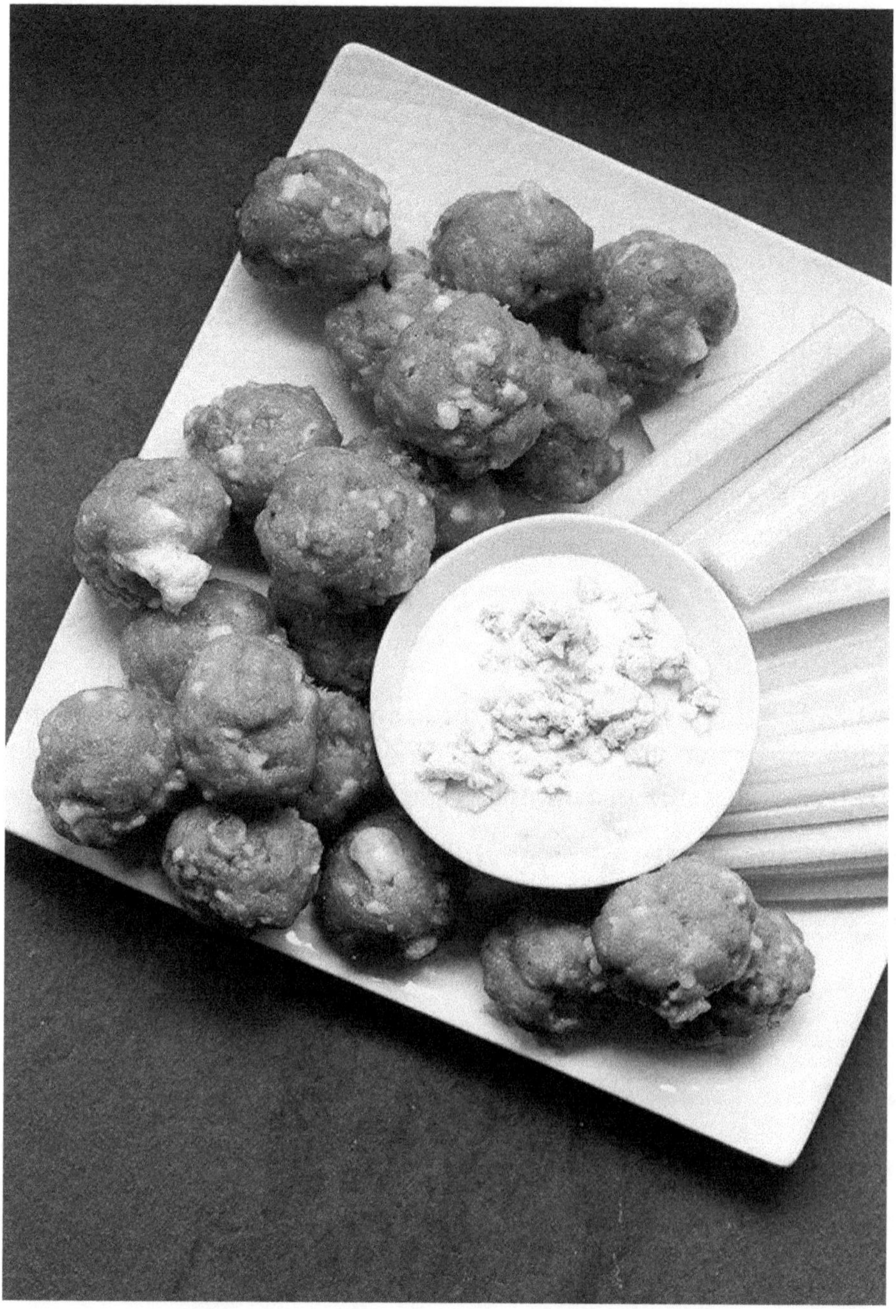

Low-Carb Smoked Salmon Blinis

Looking for an easy recipe for holiday entertaining that is also low-carb? These one-bite low carb smoked salmon blinis are the perfect snack to serve or take to your next holiday party.

Ingredients: 6 servings

- 3 eggs
- ½ cup coconut flour
- 4 oz smoked salmon
- 8 oz cream cheese
- ¾ cup milk
- ¼ cup dill sprigs, finely chopped
- ½ teaspoon gluten-free baking powder
- 4 tablespoons butter, 2 tablespoons melted and 2 tablespoons for cooking
- ½ teaspoon salt
- 1 tablespoon lemon juice

Directions:

- Mix together in a bowl, the coconut flour, baking powder and salt.
- Add the eggs and stir gently till combined.

• Pour in the melted butter (2 tablespoons).

• Now add in the milk gradually, stirring until combined after each addition.

• Continue to add the milk until it is combined and the batter is thick.

• Heat a frypan to medium heat and add a teaspoon butter.

• Using a teaspoon, add a dollop of batter to the frypan and press down with the back of the spoon to form a flat round shape. Continue to add teaspoons of batter till pan is filled.

• Cook for about 2 minutes or until browned and then flip and cook for another 1-2 minutes on the other side.

• Place cooked blinis on a plate lined with paper towel.

• Add another teaspoon butter to the pan and cook another batch of blinis. Continue until all the batter is used.

• In a bowl, combine the cream cheese with 1 tablespoon lemon juice.

• Top each blini with some of the cream cheese mixture, smoked salmon and dill.

Nutritional info per serving (5 blinis per serving): Calories 313, Fat 25g, Net Carbs 9g, Protein 10g

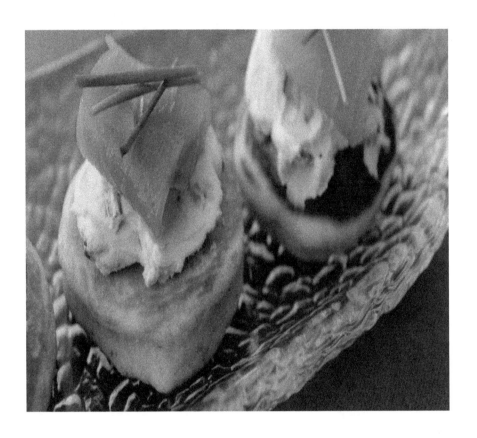

Sweet Chili Thai Chicken Wings

These delicious keto low carb sweet chili Thai chicken wings are the perfect sticky Asian chicken wings! With a homemade Thai sweet chili sauce, you won't have to worry about any added sugar or starch!

Ingredients: 3 servings

- 1 tablespoon olive oil
- 5 tablespoons Thai sweet chili sauce
- 1 teaspoon red pepper flakes
- ½ teaspoon cayenne pepper
- 1 teaspoon black pepper
- 1 teaspoon salt

Thai Sweet Chili Sauce: 12 tablespoons

- 10 tablespoons sugar-free marmelade
- 2 tablespoons coconut aminos
- 1 teaspoon paprika powder
- 2 tablespoons fish sauce
- 1 teaspoon chili oil
- ½ teaspoon tabasco
- 2 teaspoons sesame oil
- 1 teaspoon red pepper flakes

• 1 teaspoon stevia powder

Directions:

• Preheat the oven to 375 degrees F.

• If your wings include their wingtip, chop it off with a knife. Prepare the Thai sweet chili sauce recipe.

• Add the wings and drumsticks to a baking pan and drizzle the olive oil all over. Sprinkle the salt, pepper and cayenne pepper all over the wings and mix with your hands so that the spices and oil have coated all of the wings. Line them up properly on the baking tray.

• Place in the oven and bake 45 minutes.

• Take the wings out of the oven and transfer to a large frying pan. Add the Thai sweet chili sauce to the pan and coat the wings. Cook 2-5 minutes until the sauce has simmered down, thickened and coated all of the wings.

Thai Sweet Chili Sauce:

• Add all the ingredients into a bowl and mix together with a whisk or fork. The sauce is now ready to be added to any dish. Keep in the fridge for 3-4 weeks.

Nutritional info per serving: Calories 581, Fat 35.7g, Net Carbs 8.2g, Protein 56.2g

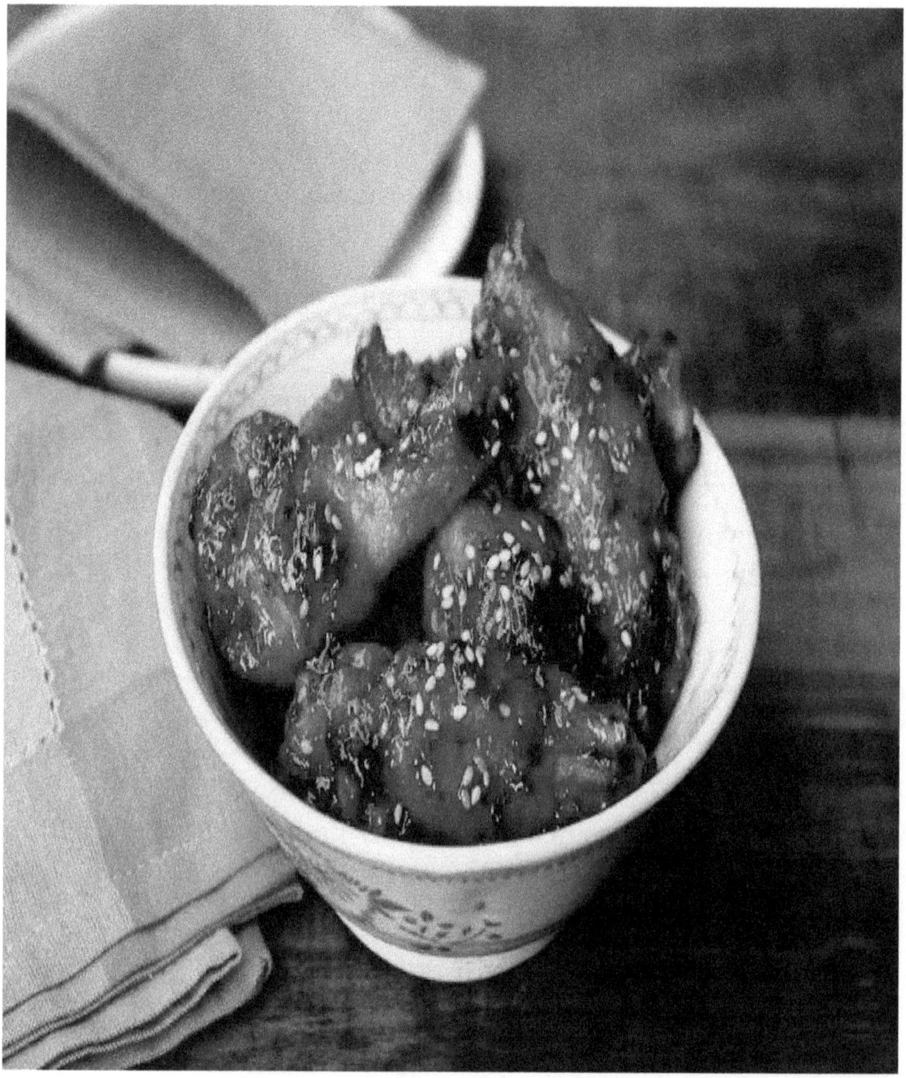

Spicy Keto Roasted Nuts

Crunchy, salty, and spicy! These keto nuts will keep you and your guests coming back for more, and more, and more!

Ingredients: 6 servings

• 8 oz pecans or almonds or walnuts

• 1 tablespoon olive oil or coconut oil

• 1 teaspoon paprika powder or chili powder

• 1 teaspoon ground cumin

• 1 teaspoon salt

Directions:

• Mix all ingredients in a medium frying pan, and cook on medium heat until the almonds are warmed through.

• Let cool and serve as a snack with a drink. Store in a container with lid at room temperature.

Nutritional info per serving: Calories 281, Fat 29g, Net Carbs 2g, Protein 4g

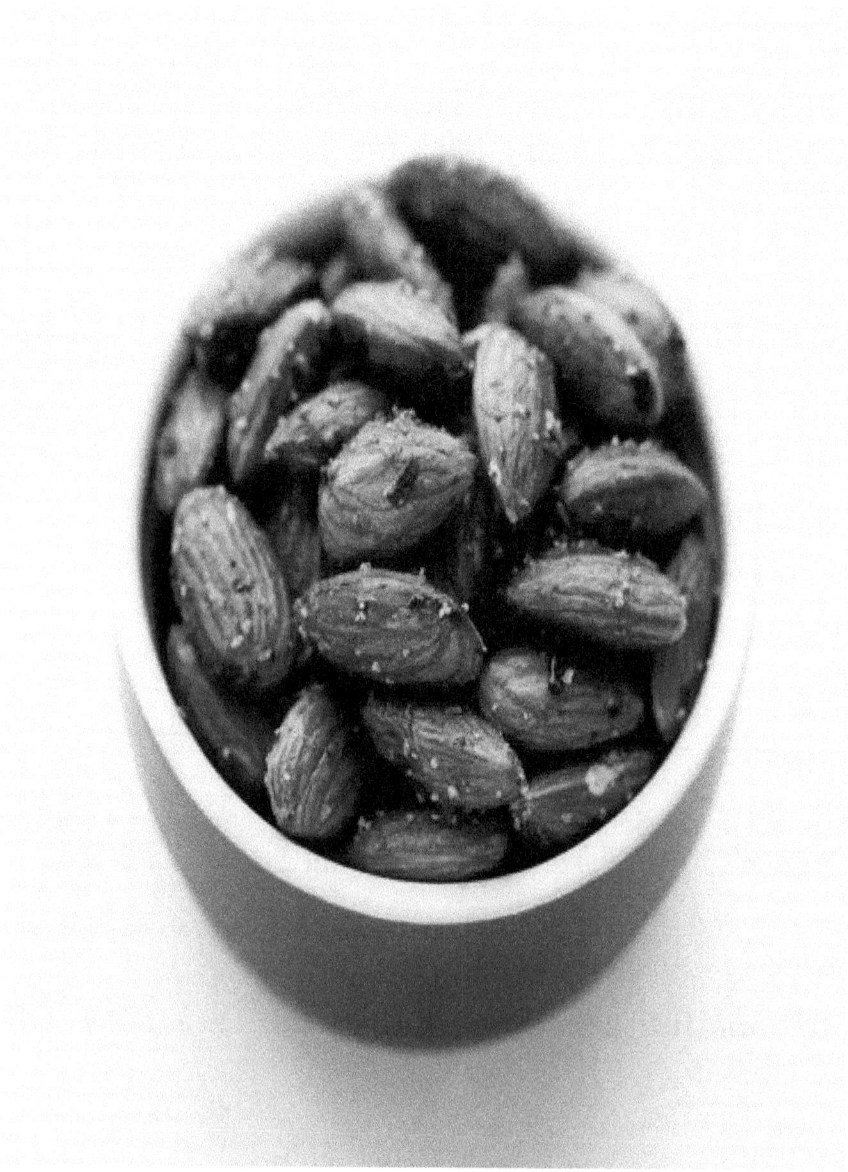

Poultry

Keto Guacamole Chicken Bacon Burgers

This keto guacamole chicken bacon burger is cut from the same cloth as those other over the top burgers but it's a lot healthier. No carb-filled, deep-fried, toppings to be found here. Just fresh flavorful guacamole packed with creamy avocado goodness, accented by tangy lime and cilantro.

Ingredients: 8 servings

For the Burgers:

- 4 chicken breasts

- 4 slices of bacon

- 2 cloves garlic

- ¼ medium onion

- 4 tablespoons avocado oil, to cook with

For the Guacamole:

- 1 large avocado, destoned and mashed

- 1 small tomato, diced

- ¼ medium onion, diced

- 2 tablespoons fresh cilantro, chopped

- 2 tablespoons lime juice

Directions:

- Food process the chicken, bacon, onion, and garlic and form patties. You might need to do this in batches.

- Fry the patties in the avocado oil in batches. Make sure the burgers are fully cooked.

- Make the guacamole by mixing together avocado, tomato, onion, lime juice, and cilantro.

- Serve the burgers with the guacamole.

Nutritional info per serving: Calories 364, Fat 27g, Net Carbs 2g, Protein 26g

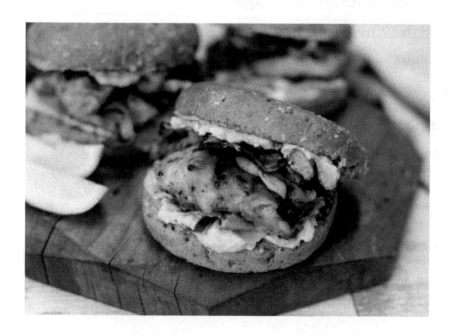

Holiday Turkey with Low-Carb Stuffing and Gravy

Be prepared to wow family and friends with this turkey! It's loaded with fresh citrus flavor, and the earthy tones of sage. And the orange butter makes the meat unbelievably moist and juice.

Ingredients: 12 servings

Turkey:

- 12 lbs turkey

- 10 oz celery root, roughly chopped

- 2 tablespoons olive oil

- 2 yellow onions, finely chopped

- 2 carrots, roughly chopped

- 1 orange, juiced

- giblets from the turkey

- 1 cup water

- 1 teaspoon ground black pepper

- 2 teaspoons kosher salt or ground sea salt

Orange and Sage Butter:

- 10 oz butter, at room temperature

- 2-3 fresh sage sprigs, finely chopped

- 2 shallots, finely chopped
- 1 orange, the zest
- 1 teaspoon kosher salt or ground sea salt
- ¼ teaspoon ground black pepper

Stuffing:

- 3 tablespoons butter
- 5 1/3 bacon, diced
- ½ lb celery root, diced
- 2 pieces of low-carb bread
- 2 yellow onions, finely chopped
- 1 apple, grated
- 2 oz pecans, chopped
- 30 oz ground pork
- 2-3 fresh sage sprigs, finely chopped
- ½ teaspoon ground nutmeg
- 1 cup heavy whipping cream
- ½ teaspoon ground black pepper
- 1 teaspoon kosher salt or ground sea salt

Gravy:

- 1-2 cups juices from roasting the turkey
- 1-2 cups heavy whipping cream
- 3 oz cream cheese

Directions:

Stuffing:

• Crumble or tear the bread into pieces in a large bowl, and pour the cream on top. Let the bread absorb the cream for a few minutes.

• Sautè pork with bacon until cooked through.

• Add onion, and celery root to the pan with 2 tablespoons butter. Cook until vegetables are softened, about 5-7 minutes. Stir in the grated apple, sage, nutmeg, salt, pepper, and pecans.

• Stir bread into the mixture.

• Set aside and let cool.

• Butter a baking dish with the remaining butter. Reserve 1/3 stuffing mixture to stuff the turkey. Place the rest in the prepared baking dish, and refrigerate until 30 minutes before the turkey is done.

• Bake until browned and crunchy, about 25-30 minutes.

Butter and Turkey:

• In a medium bowl, combine all of the orange butter ingredients.

• Using your fingers, gently loosen the breast skin and push in the orange butter. A good place to start is around the neck and thighs.

• Spread butter under the turkey breast and thighs.

• Reserve a third of the seasoned butter.

• Pat the turkey dry with paper towels. Remove the giblets, and reserve.

• Salt and pepper the turkey. Tie together the thighs with cotton cooking string. Place the turkey in a big roasting pan, breast up.

Tuck the wings under the turkey so that they won't dry out during roasting. Stuff a third of the stuffing mix into the turkey.

• Preheat the oven to 350 degrees F. Place root vegetables, onion and giblets around the turkey. Salt and pepper and add olive oil on top of the vegetables. Sprinkle the sage on top. Add one cup of water.

• Place the rest of the orange butter on top of the turkey. Cover with squeezed orange juice. Roughly chop the orange into wedges, and add to pan.

• Place a piece of aluminum foil on the breast part to protect it from drying out. Place on lower rack in the oven and roast the turkey for 3 ½ - 4 ½ hours. Baste the turkey every hour with pan juices. One hour before the turkey is done, remove the aluminum foil to allow the breast skin to roast.

• Remove from the oven. Transfer the turkey to a large cutting board or serving plate. Tent with aluminum foil for 15-20 minutes, before serving.

Gravy:

• Remove the vegetables and giblets from the baking pan. Pour the cooking juices through a strainer into a saucepan. Bring to a boil and reduce by 30-40%. Season with salt and pepper to taste.

• Add heavy cream and cream cheese. Bring to a boil and lower the heat. Let simmer until desired consistency.

Nutritional info per serving: Calories 1413, Fat 96g, Net Carbs 14g, Protein 118g

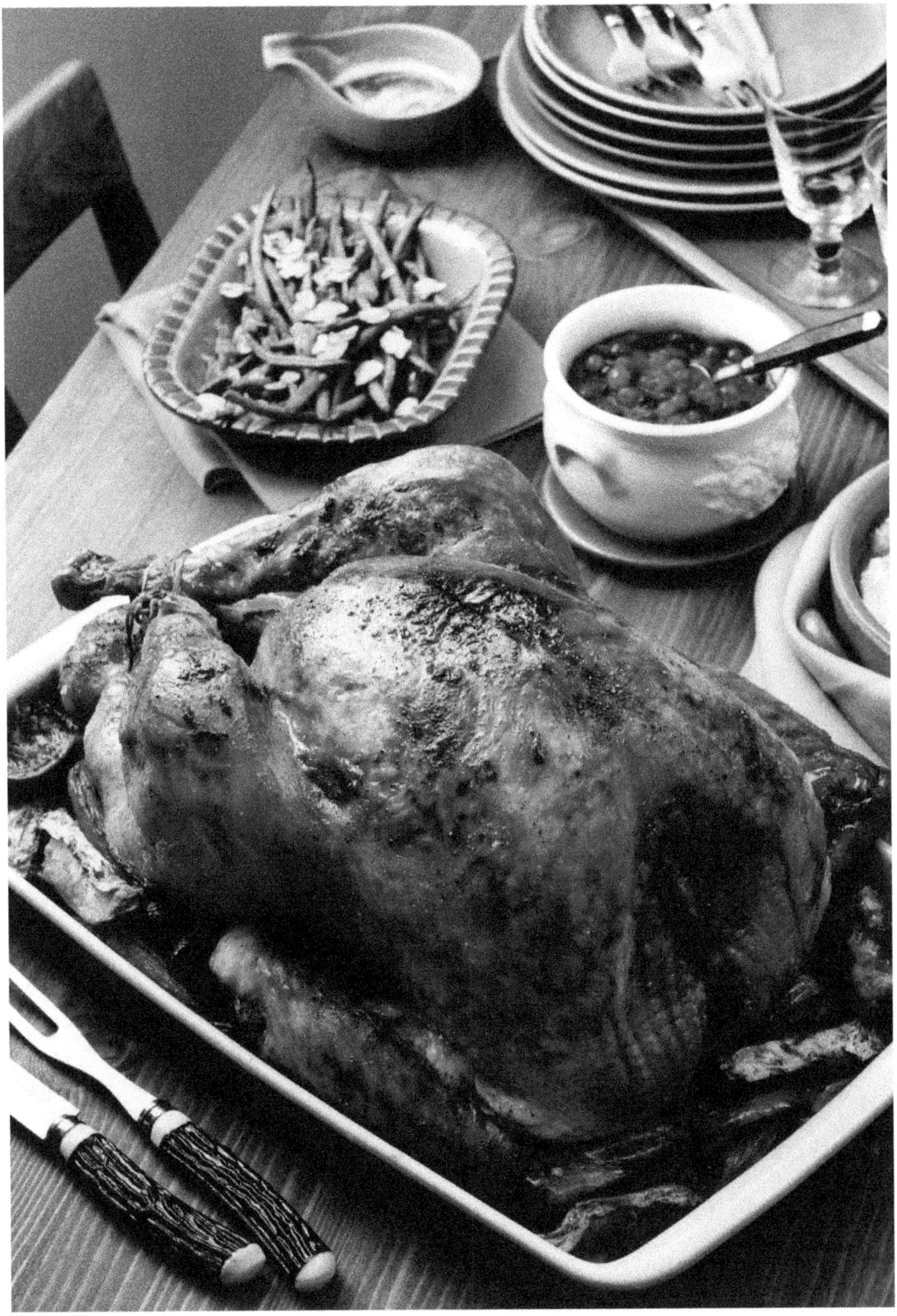

Asian Keto Chicken Thighs

This Asian keto chicken thighs recipe is easy to make and enjoyable to eat! Chicken thighs are very flavorful, and cooking with the skin on will give them a nice flavor boost from the fat.

Ingredients: 4 servings

• 8 chicken thighs, skin on

• ½ cup tamari sauce

• ½ onion, sliced

• 4 cloves garlic, minced

• ¼ cup water

• 1 teaspoon sesame seeds, for garnish

• 1 green onion, chopped for garnish

• Salt and pepper, to taste

Directions:

• Place the chicken thighs at the bottom of the pot.

• Then add in the sliced onions, tamari sauce, garlic, and water. Try to cover most of the chicken in the sauce.

• Set on low heat for 6 hours.

• Season with salt and pepper to taste.

• Garnish with chopped green onions and sesame seeds.

• Roast the thighs in the oven on a baking tray for 15-20 minutes to brown and crisp up the skin.

Nutritional info per serving: Calories 434, Fat 29g, Net Carbs 4g, Protein 32g

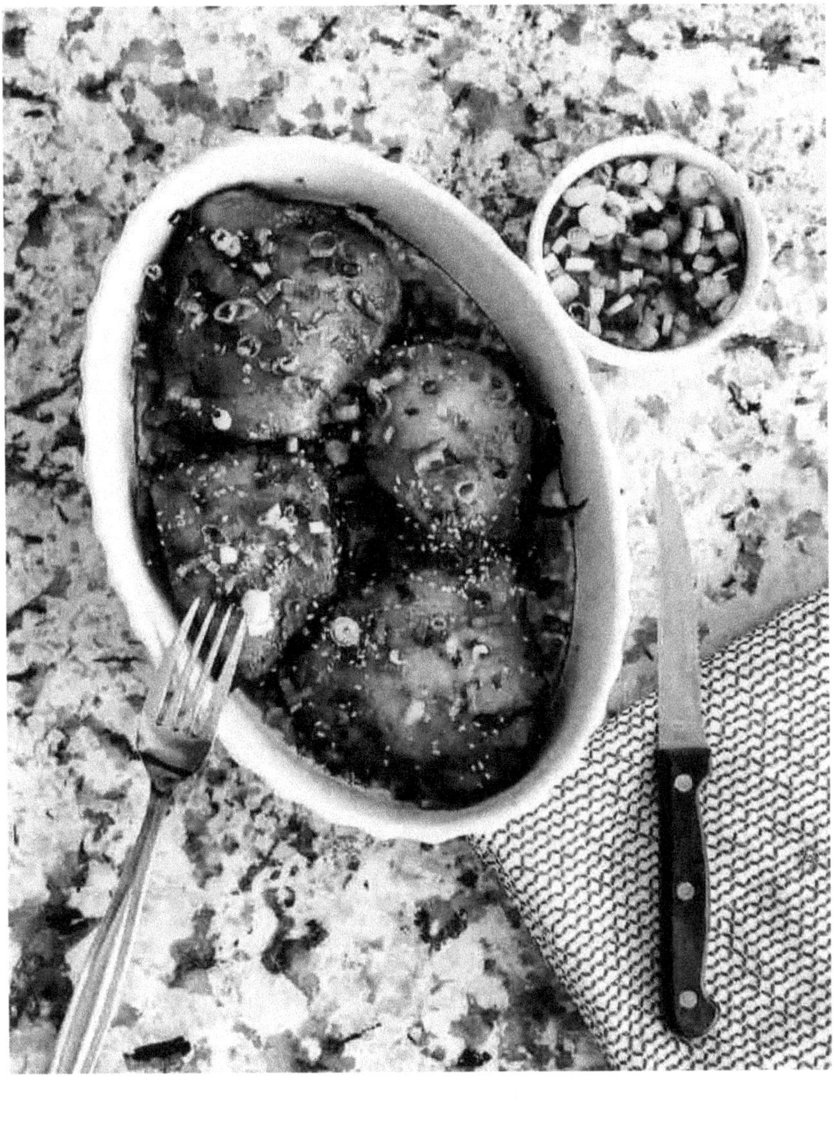

Roast Quail with Rosemary, Thyme and Garlic

Such a simple dish, yet impressive! A few quails seasoned with herb butter and roast in the oven. That's all it takes to put a stunning main course on the table.

Ingredients: 4 servings

- 8 whole quail, washed, dried with paper towel
- 2 fresh thyme sprigs, leaves picked
- 8 cloves garlic, peeled and bruised
- 2 tablespoons butter, cubed
- 1 small lemon, cut into eighths
- 1 fresh rosemary sprig, leaves picked
- ½ cup massel chicken style liquid stock
- Steamed waxy potatoes, to serve
- ¼ cup dry white wine
- Green beans, to serve
- Salt and ground black pepper, to taste

Herb Butter:

- 3 tablespoons butter, at room temperature
- 1 tablespoon fresh rosemary leaves, finely chopped
- 2 tablespoons fresh thyme leaves, finely chopped

- 2 large cloves garlic, crushed

- Salt and ground black pepper, to taste

Directions:

- Preheat the oven to 390 degrees F.

- To make the herb butter, place the butter, thyme, garlic, rosemary, salt and pepper in a small bowl and mix well to combine.

- Use your fingers to carefully loosen the skin over the quail breasts. Spread herb butter over the breasts and then re-cover with the skin.

- Divide the lemon, butter, thyme, garlic and rosemary among the cavities of the quail. Tie the legs together with wet unwaxed string.

- Place the quail in a single layer in a large roasting pan. Roast in preheated oven for 35 minutes or until the juices are pale pink when a fine skewer is inserted into the thigh. Remove the quail from the roasting pan and place on a large plate. Cover loosely with foil and stand for 10 minutes to rest.

- Meanwhile, place roasting pan over medium heat. Add the stock and white wine and cook for 1 minute, scraping with a wooden spoon to dislodge any residue left on the base of the pan. Bring to a boil and simmer, uncovered, for 2-3 minutes or until reduced by ½. Taste and season with salt and pepper.

- Serve the quail with the sauce, potatoes and beans.

Nutritional info per serving: Calories 1194, Fat 26g, Net Carbs 2g, Protein 10g

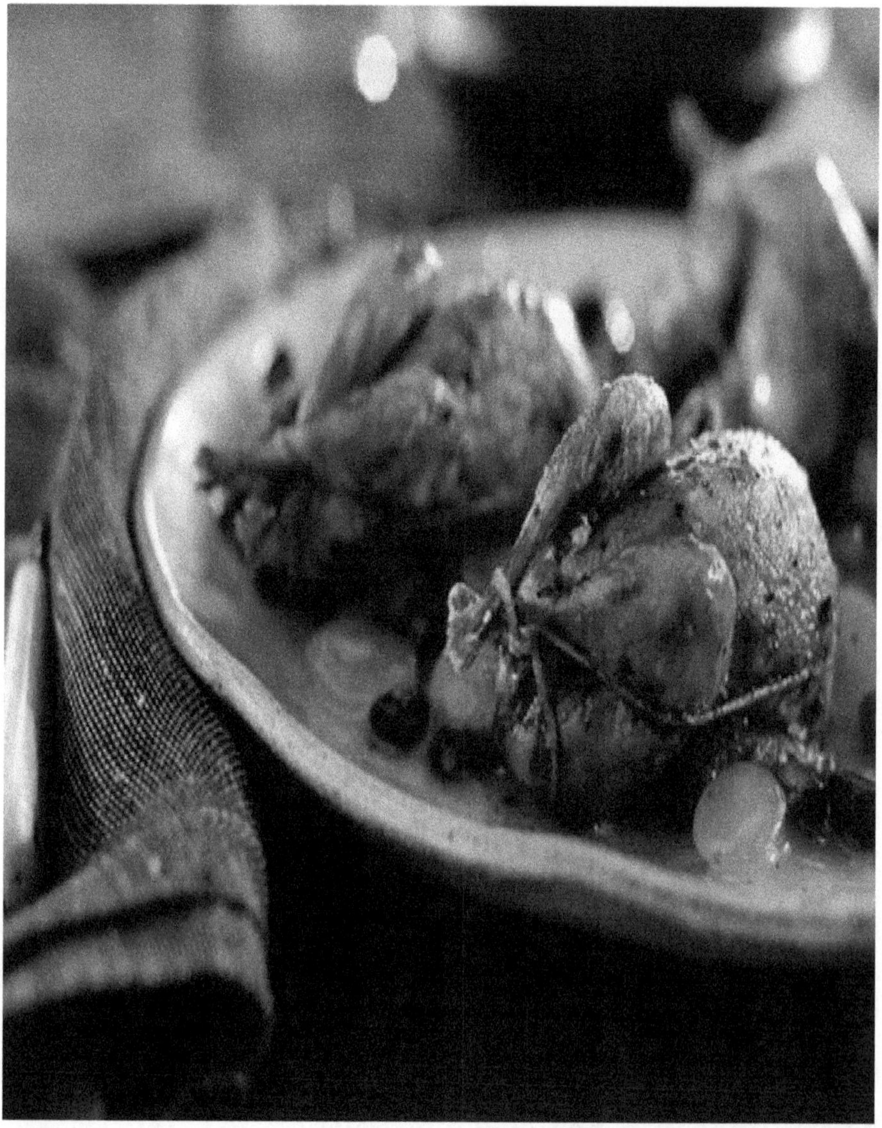

Keto Chicken Fajita Bowl

Need a simple, vibrant midweek meal the family will love? This recipe is quick, simple and tasty with minimal clean up. Have it both ways. A warm and satisfying meal, and a fresh salad, rolled into one.

Ingredients: 4 servings

- 1 ½ lbs boneless chicken thighs
- 10 oz Romaine lettuce
- 2 avocados
- 2 tablespoons Tex-Mex seasoning
- 5 oz Mexican cheese
- 5 oz cherry tomatoes
- 4 tablespoons fresh cilantro
- 1 yellow onion
- 1 green bell pepper
- 3 oz butter
- 1 cup sour cream
- Salt and pepper, to taste

Directions:

• Prepare the toppings: Tear the lettuce, chop tomatoes, dice avocados, and clean and chop the cilantro. Grate the cheese if not pre-shredded. Set aside.

• Slice onion and pepper fairly thin.

• On a separate cutting board, cut the chicken into thin strips.

• Fry the chicken in butter in a large skillet over medium/high heat. Salt and pepper to taste. When the chicken is almost cooked through, add onion, pepper and Tex-Mex seasoning.

• Lower the heat and continue to fry while stirring for a couple of minutes until the chicken is thoroughly cooked and the vegetables have softened just a bit.

• Place lettuce in a bowl and add the chicken mixture. Add shredded cheese, diced avocado, chopped tomatoes, fresh cilantro and a dollop of sour cream.

Nutritional info per serving: Calories 862, Fat 71g, Net Carbs 9g, Protein 41g

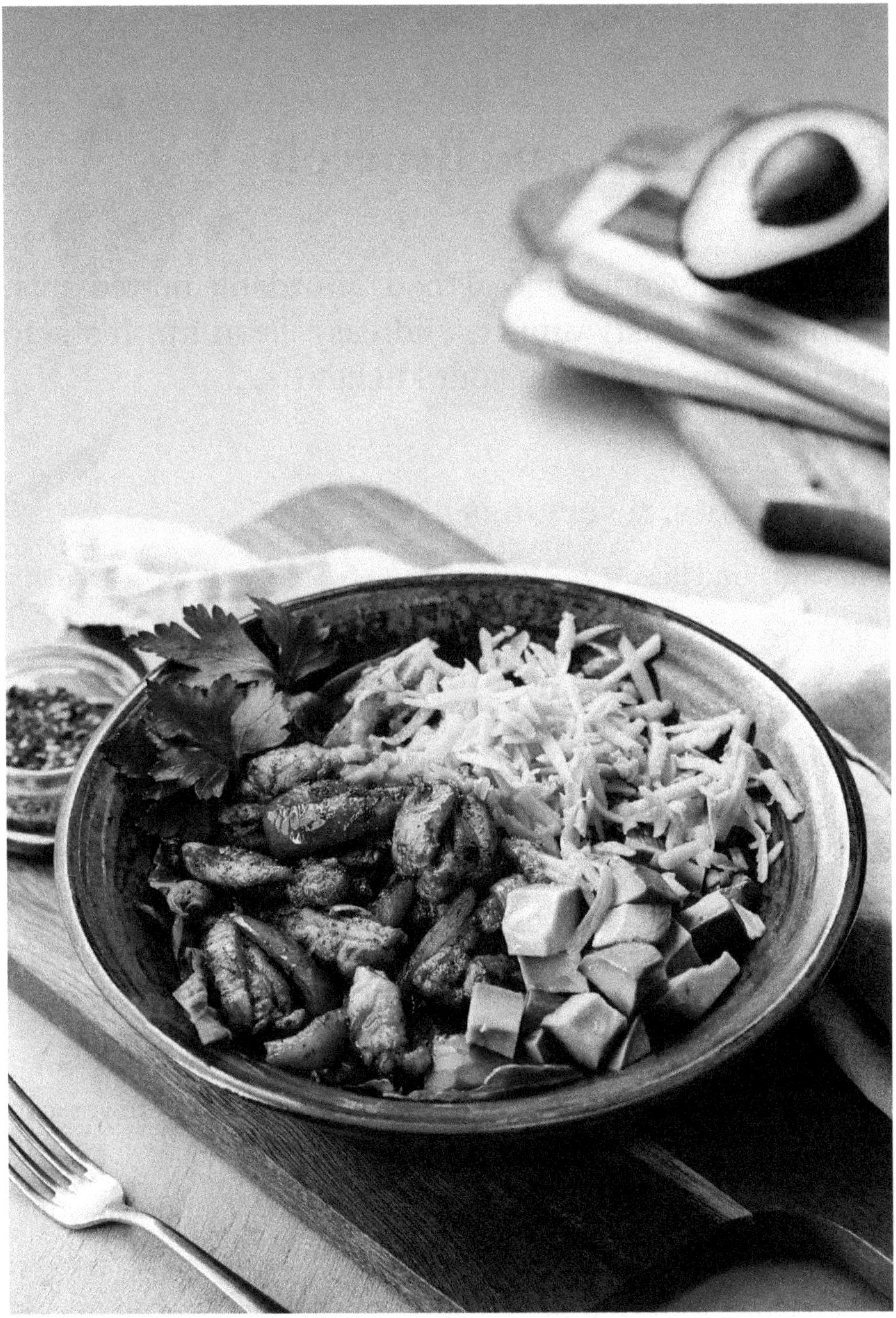

Meat

Ground Beef and Broccoli

A one-skillet wonder! Real food, affordable ingredients, simple prep, tasty dinner, and easy clean up. It's keto fast food, made right in your kitchen!

Ingredients: 2 servings

- 10 oz ground beef
- 9 oz broccoli
- 3 oz butter
- ½ cup mayonnaise or crème fraìche
- Salt and pepper, to taste

Directions:

• Rinse and trim the broccoli, including the stem. Cut into small florets. Peel the stem and cut into small pieces.

• Heat up a hearty dollop of butter in a frying pan where you can fit both the ground beef and broccoli.

• Brown the ground beef on high heat until it's almost done. Season with salt and pepper to taste.

• Lower the heat. Add more butter and fry the broccoli for 3-5 minutes. Stir the ground beef every now and then.

• Season the broccoli. Top with the remaining butter and serve while still hot. It's also delicious to serve with an extra dollop of crème fraîche or mayonnaise.

Nutritional info per serving: Calories 648, Fat 54g, Net Carbs 5g, Protein 33g

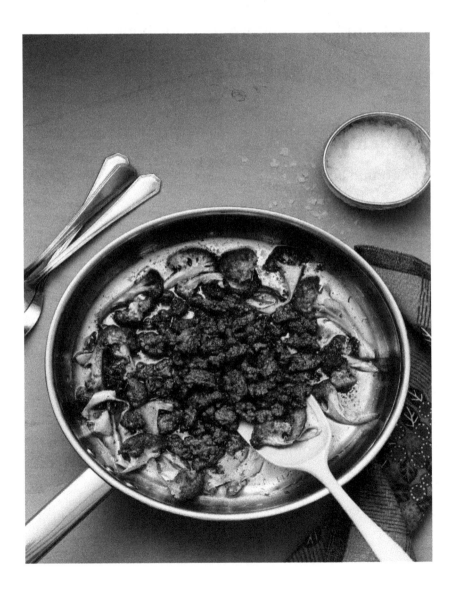

Keto Tex-Mex Casserole

Hearty and spicy like you daydream about. Loaded with classic Tex-Mex goodness, minus the carbs, this easy keto casserole will satisfy all your south-of-the-border cravings. And say goodbye to store-bought guacamole and packaged taco seasoning! Making your own is simple, healthy and delicious.

Ingredients: 4 servings

- 25 oz ground beef
- 3 tablespoons Tex-Mex seasoning
- 2 oz butter
- 7 oz shredded cheese
- 7 oz crushed tomatoes
- 2 oz pickled jalapenos

Serving:

- 1 cup guacamole
- 1 scallion, finely chopped
- 1 cup crème fraìche or sour cream
- 5 oz leafy greens or iceberg lettuce

Directions:

• Preheat the oven to 400 degrees F.

• Fry the ground beef in butter on medium/high heat, until cooked through and no longer pink.

• Add Tex-Mex seasoning and crushed tomatoes. Stir and let simmer for 5 minutes. Taste to see if it needs additional salt and pepper.

• Place the ground beef mixture in a greased baking dish. Top with jalapeno and cheese.

• Bake on upper rack in the oven for 15-20 minutes or until golden brown on top.

• Chop the scallion finely and mix with the crème fraîche or sour cream in a separate bowl.

• Serve the casserole warm with a dollop of the crème fraîche or sour cream, guacamole and a green salad.

Nutritional info per serving: Calories 870, Fat 70 g, Net Carbs 8g, Protein 50g

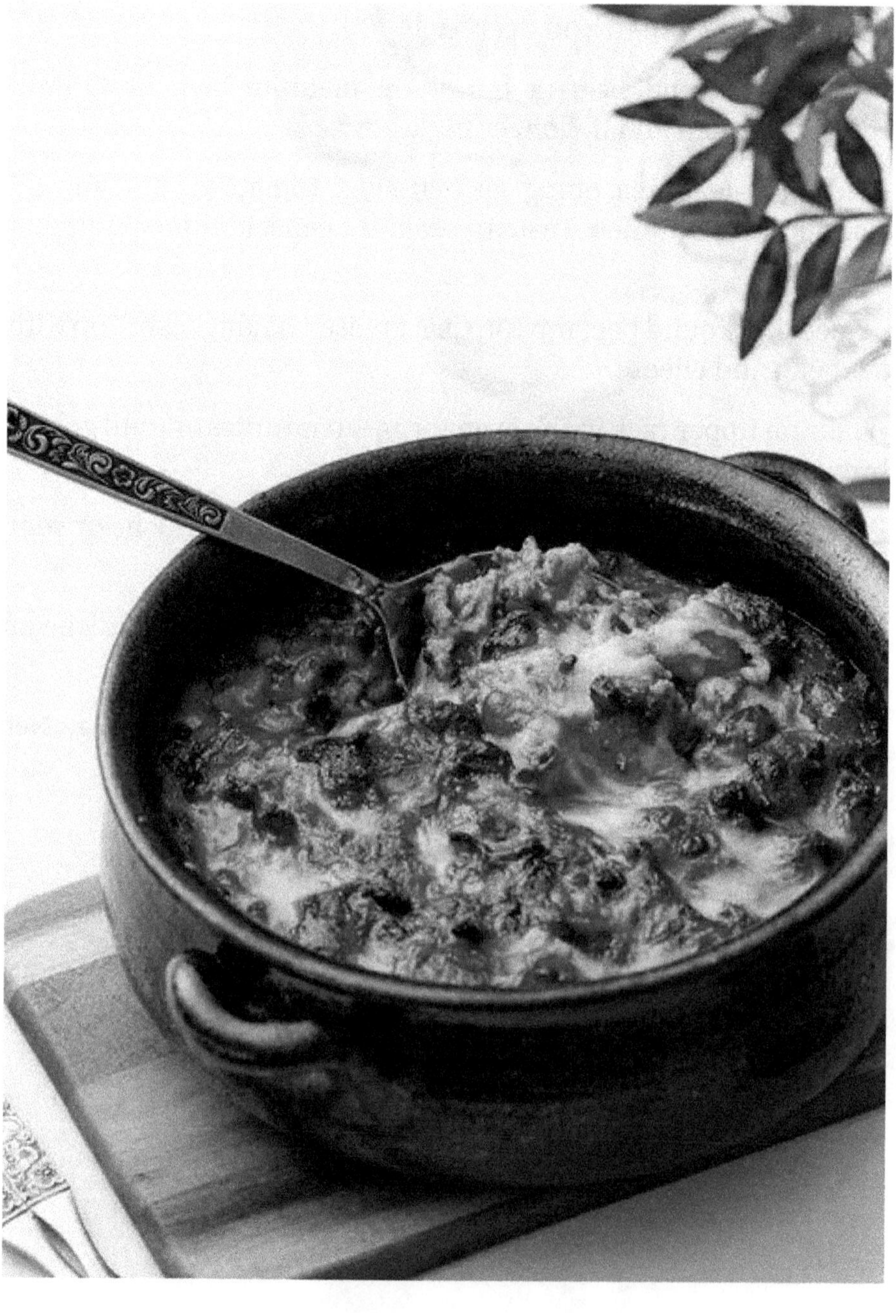

Easy Zucchini Beef Sautè with Garlic and Cilantro

If you're looking for a fast and nutritious meal, then this is a great recipe for you! It's super fast because the beef and the zucchini are chopped into thin strips so that they cook quickly, and it's delicious because the garlic, cilantro, and gluten-free tamari soy sauce add tons of flavor to the dish.

Ingredients: 2 servings

- 10 oz beef, sliced into 1-2 inch strips
- 1 zucchini, cut into 1-2 inch long thin strips
- ¼ cup cilantro, chopped
- 3 cloves garlic, minced or diced
- Avocado oil, to cook with
- 2 tablespoons gluten-free tamari sauce

Directions:

- Place 2 tablespoons of avocado oil into a frying pan on high heat.
- Add the the strips of beef into the frying pan and saute for a few minutes on high heat.
- When the beef is browned, add in the zucchini strips and keep sauteing.

• When the zucchini is soft, add in the tamari sauce, garlic, and cilantro.

• Saute for a few minutes more and serve immediately.

Nutritional info per serving: Calories 304, Fat 40g, Net Carbs 5g, Protein 31g

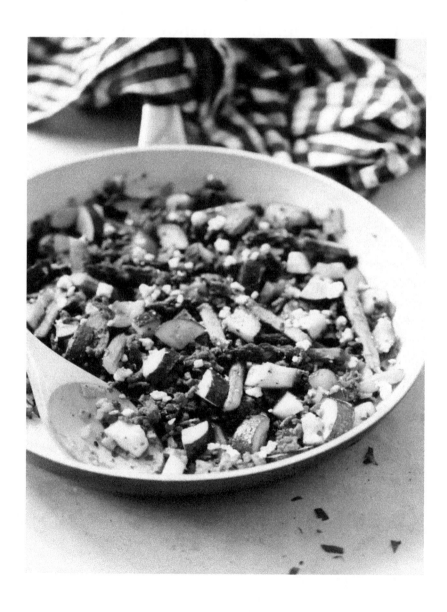

Pork Egg Roll in a Bowl

Pork egg roll in a bowl is a delicious dish with Asian flavor. The main vegetables in this recipe are cabbage, red bell peppers, onion and celery.

Ingredients: 4 servings

- 1 lb ground pork
- 5 cups cabbage, shredded
- 3 celery stalks, small size
- 2 cloves garlic, minced
- ½ onion, small size
- ½ red bell pepper
- 2 tablespoons sesame oil
- ½ teaspoon chili powder
- 1 teaspoon ground ginger
- 2 tablespoons coconut aminos
- 1 tablespoon white vinegar
- 2 tablespoons toasted sesame seeds
- Salt and black pepper, to taste

Directions:

- After washing the celery, cabbage leaves, onion, and red pepper, transfer to individual bowls. Remove the onion skin and chop into slivers. Scoop out the seeds from the pepper and chop into ribbons as well. Throw away the celery leaves and cut the stalk lengthwise to create lean sticks. Finally, chop the cabbage leaves into fine pieces. Reserve the vegetable bowls.

• Heat oil in a wok or a large frying pan if a wok is unavailable. Fry the ground pork in the heated oil. Toss in the minced garlic, chili powder, and grated ginger. Adjust the taste with some salt and pepper. Gently pour vinegar and coconut aminos into the pan. Keep stirring for 3 minutes to separate the pork pieces apart and cook the meat faster.

• Throw in all the chopped veggies into the cooked beef. Fold altogether to mix. Stir continuously to season the veggies with the meat broth and to brown the veggies a bit.

• Top with the toasted sesame seeds. Add more salt and black pepper as necessary. Turn off the heat so as not to overcook the vegetables. Garnish with freshly chopped spring onion or coriander. Serve in a bowl.

Nutritional info per serving: Calories 427, Fat 33.5g, Net Carbs 6g, Protein 22.4g

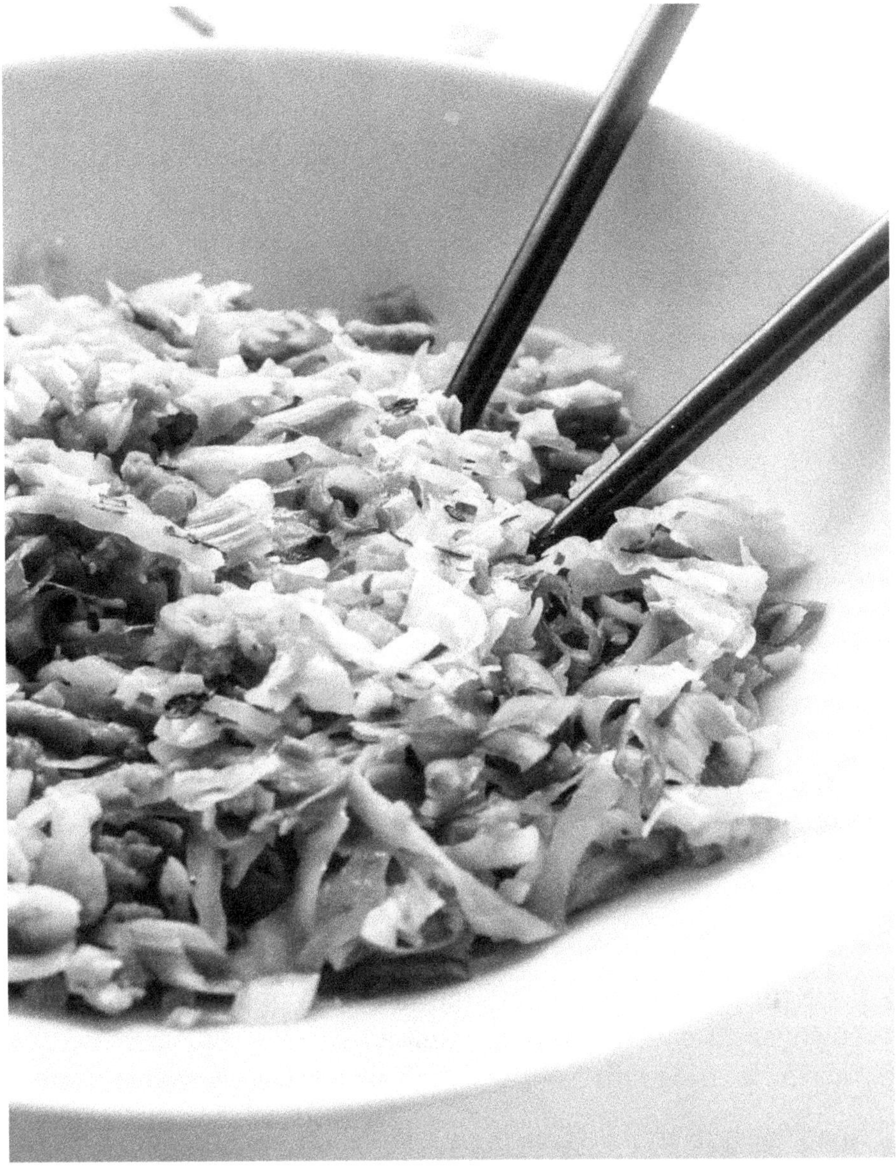

Garlic and Rosemary Grilled Lamb Chops

Grilled lamb chops infused with rosemary and garlic flavors! This delicious dish is super easy to make!

Ingredients: 4 servings

• 2 pounds lamb loin

• 4 cloves garlic, minced

• 1 tablespoon fresh rosemary, chopped

• ¼ cup olive oil

• Zest of 1 lemon

• ½ teaspoon ground black pepper

• 1 ¼ teaspoon kosher salt

Directions:

• Combine the garlic, rosemary, lemon zest, olive oil, salt and pepper in a measuring cup.

• Pour the marinade over the lamb chops, making sure to flip them over to cover them completely. Cover and marinate the chops in the fridge for as little as 1 hour, or as long as overnight.

• Heat the grill to medium/high heat, then sear the lamb chops for 2-3 minutes, on each side. Lower the heat to medium then cook them for 5-6 minutes, or until the internal temperature reads 150 degrees F.

• Allow the lamb chops to rest on a plate covered with aluminum foil for 5 minutes before serving.

Nutritional info per serving: Calories 172, Fat 7.8g, Net Carbs 0.4g, Protein 23.2g

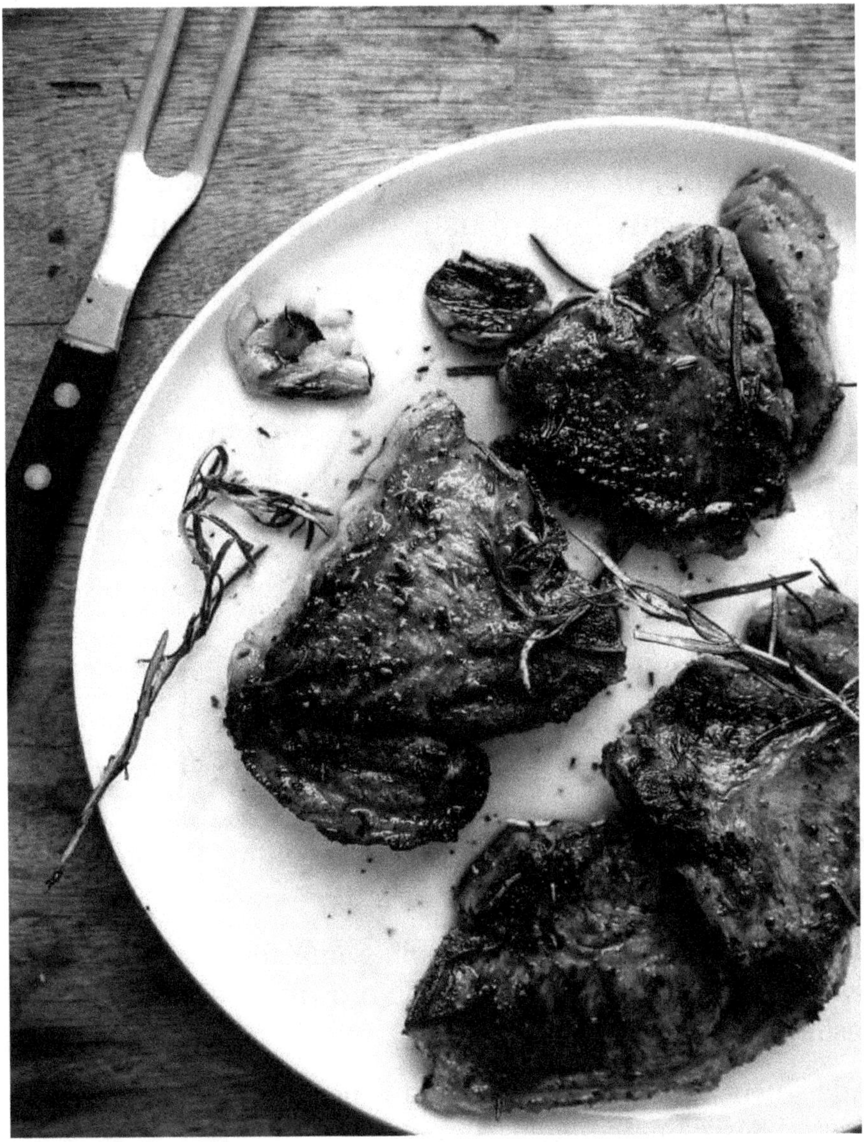

Veggies & Sides

Butter-Fried Broccoli

Ready to give broccoli a make-over of epic proportions? So simple yet profound, the answer is butter! Fry up the broccoli alone, or with scallions and capers. Serve with eggs, meat or any kind of fish. In a word: Fabulous!

Ingredients: 4 servings

- 15 oz broccoli
- 3 oz butter
- 5 scallions
- 2 tablespoons small capers
- Salt and pepper

Directions:

• Divide the broccoli into small florets, including the stem. Peel the stem if it is rough.

• Melt the butter and add broccoli. Sautè for 5 minutes over medium/high heat until the broccoli browns nicely and softens. Season with salt and pepper.

• Add finely chopped scallions and capers. Fry for another 1-2 minutes. Serve immediately.

Nutritional info per serving: Calories 202, Fat 19g, Net Carbs 5g, Protein 3g

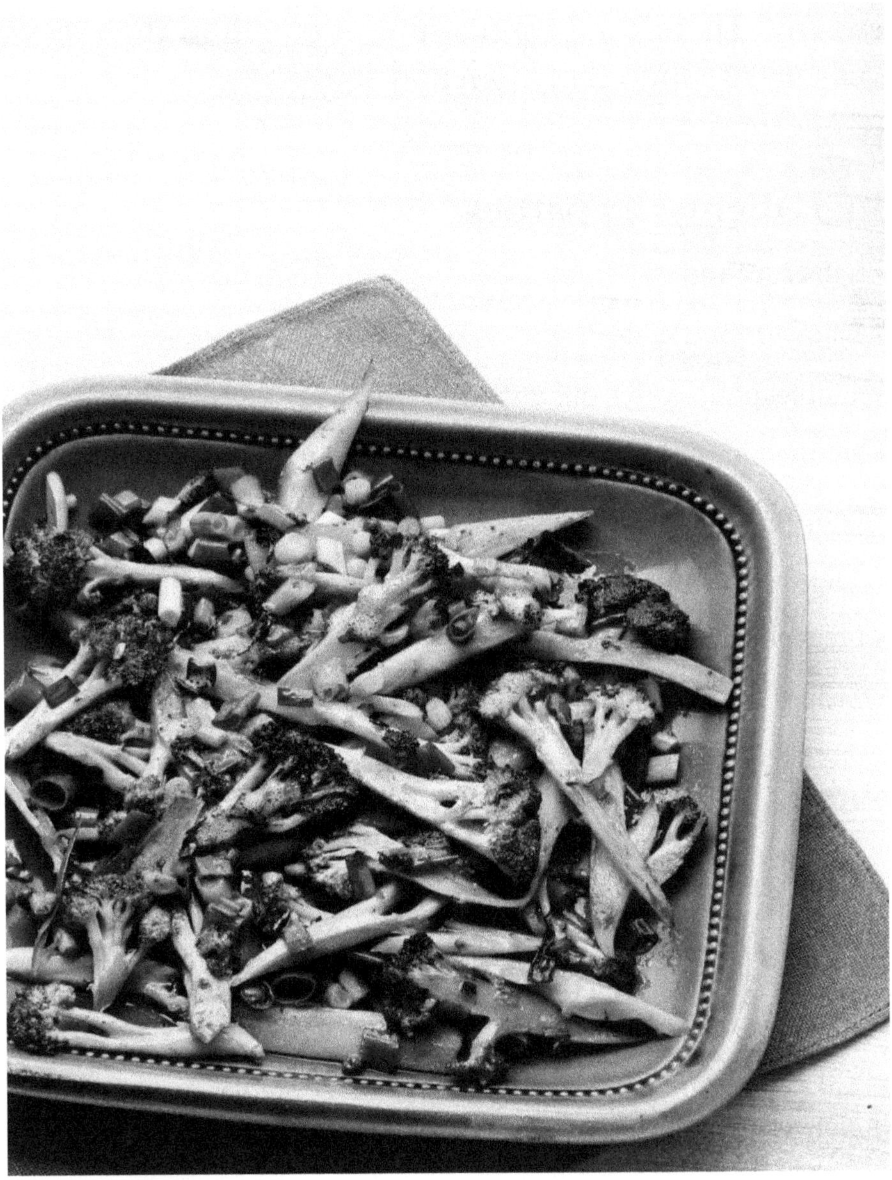

Creamy Greek Zucchini Patties

These creamy Greek zucchini patties are so delicious! I've labeled as "creamy" because they are so incredibly creamy. There's not even a hint of cream in the recipe, yet they are incredibly rich and soft.

Ingredients: 24 patties

• 2 lbs zucchini

• 1 cup almond meal

• 3 tablespoons olive oil, divided

• 2 large handfuls fresh herbs (mint, dill and parsley)

• 1 cup crumbled feta cheese

• 2 large free-range organic eggs

• 1 teaspoon ground cumin

• Ground black pepper to taste

• 1 teaspoon fine grain sea salt

Directions:

• Wash zucchini and cut off the ends. Grate them on the side holes of a grates. Place grated zucchini in a colander and sprinkle with salt. Leave to drain for at least 10 minutes (1 hour best).

• Take handfuls of the zucchini and squeeze out all of the moisture.

• In a large bowl, beat the eggs, add grated zucchini, herbs, cumin, almond meal, feta, salt and pepper. Mix together well.

• Transfer mixture to the refrigerator for 20 minutes to allow the almond meal to suck up some of the moisture.

• Take small handfuls of mixture and form into patties. If it seems wet, add more almond meal, one tablespoon at a time.

• Heat one tablespoon of olive oil in a large nonstick frying pan over medium/high heat. When hot, cook the patties in batches until golden brown, about 5 minutes per side.

• Remove and drain briefly on paper towel to soak up any excess grease. Serve.

Nutritional info per serving (1 patty): Calories 53, Fat 5g, Net Carbs 2g, Protein 2g

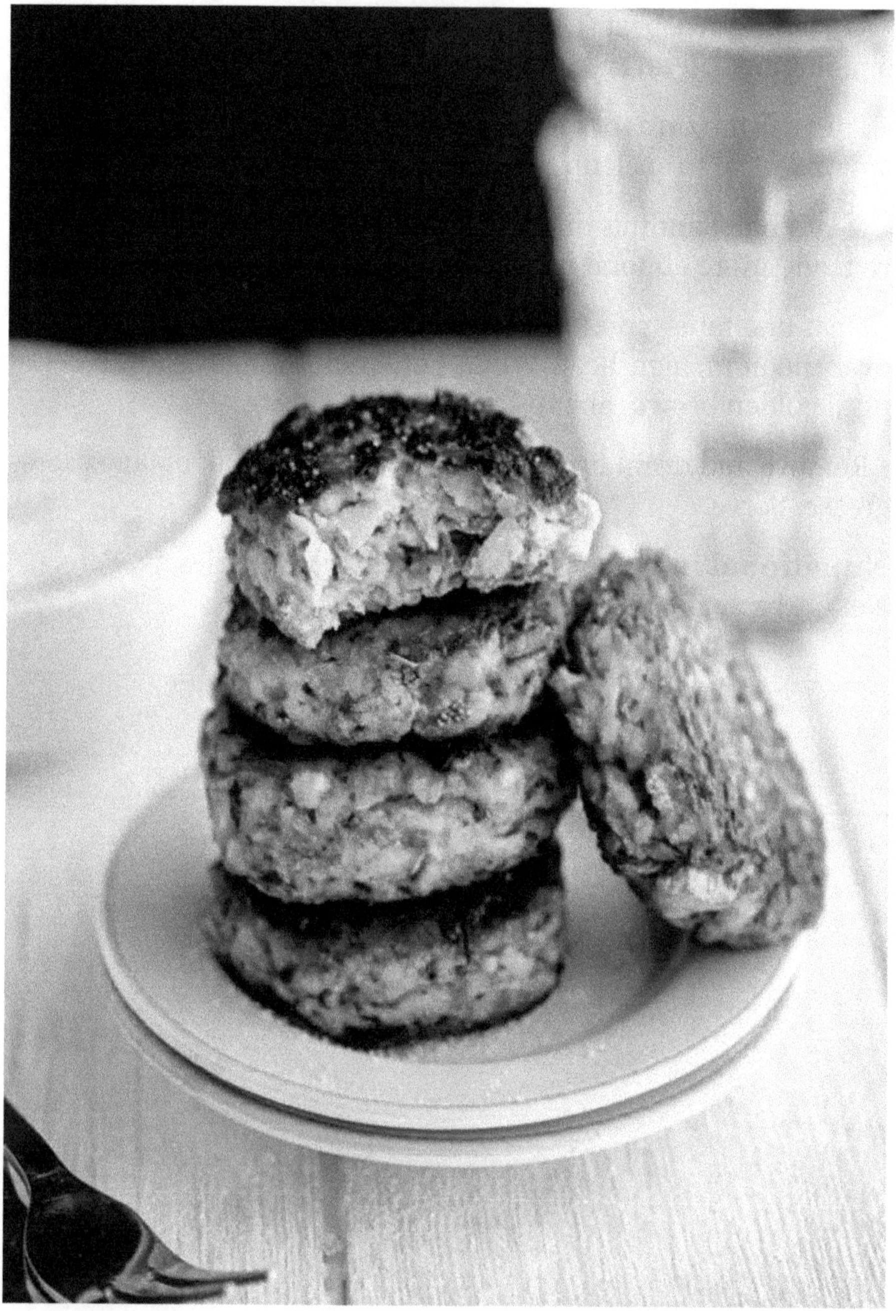

Parmesan Brussels Sprouts

Healthy and tasty! You can make these Parmesan brussels sprouts into a vegetarian main by stirring through some cooked quinoa or bulgur wheat!

Ingredients: 8 servings

• 2 lbs brussel sprouts

• 2 tablespoons extra virgin olive oil

• 4 tablespoons freshly grated Parmesan cheese

• 1 lemon

• 1 teaspoon chili flakes

• Zest of half lemon

• Black pepper

• Pinch of sea salt

Directions:

• Preheat the oven to 430 degrees F.

• Trim and halve the brussels sprouts, then place on a large baking tray. Add the oil, grate over the lemon zest, then sprinkle with the chili flakes and a pinch of sea salt and black pepper. Mix with your hands to coat.

• Roast in the oven for 10 minutes. The sprouts should start caramelise in places. When that happens, scatter over the Parmesan cheese and roast for a further 15 minutes, until the cheese is crisp and golden brown, and the sprouts tender.

Nutritional info per serving: Calories 149, Fat 8.7g, Net Carbs 5.3g, Protein 9.7g

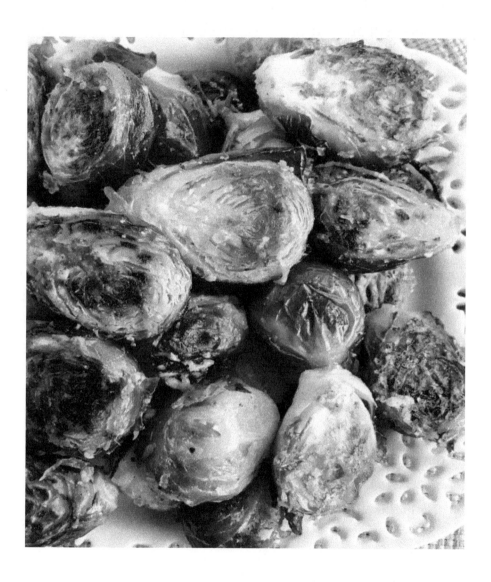

Indian Spiced Cauliflower Rice

This Indian spiced cauliflower rice is a quick, easy and wonderfully nutritious alternative to regular rice!

Ingredients: 4 servings

• 1 cauliflower, leaves and stalk removed

• 1 tablespoon coconut oil

• 1 teaspoon turmeric

• 1 teaspoon cumin

• 2 tablespoons fresh coriander, chopped roughly

• Salt and pepper to taste

Directions:

• Start by finely chopping the cauliflower.

• Heat the oil gently in a frying pan for 30 seconds, then add the spices and cook for another 30 seconds.

• Add the finely chopped cauliflower and stir fry over medium heat for 3-5 minutes until cooked to your liking.

• Stir through some salt and pepper and the fresh coriander and serve with your favorite curry.

Nutritional info per serving: Calories 64, Fat 3.5g, Net Carbs 4.3g, Protein 3g

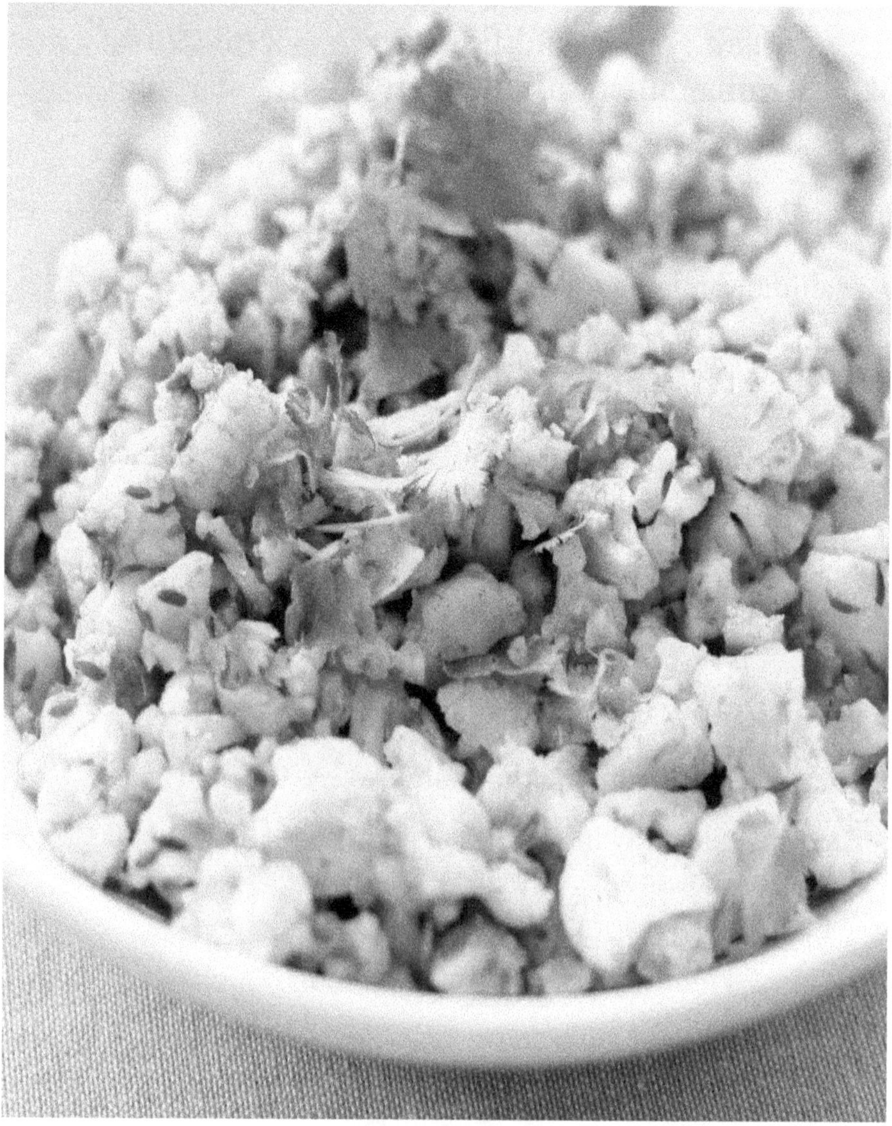

Keto Roasted Radishes

You'll fall in love with these keto roasted radishes! They are tossed with avocado oil and sprinkled with Parmesan cheese, making them the perfect low-carb keto friendly side dish!

Ingredients: 6 servings

- 1 lb raw radishes, halved

- 2 tablespoons avocado oil

- ½ cup shredded Parmesan cheese

- ¼ teaspoon ground thyme

- 1 tablespoon dried rosemary

- ¼ teaspoon pepper

- ¾ teaspoon salt

Directions:

• Preheat the oven to 450 degrees F and line a baking sheet with parchment paper.

• To a small bowl, add radishes, avocado oil, ground thyme, dried rosemary, salt, and pepper and toss using tongs or spoon until radishes are coated in oil and spices. Transfer radishes to the prepared baking sheet and bake until golden brown and crispy, about 35 minutes, flipping halfway through.

• Remove baking sheet from the oven, sprinkle radishes with Parmesan cheese, and return pan to oven to bake until cheese melts just slightly, about an additional 2-3 minutes. Remove pan from oven, garnish with fresh parsley and serve.

Nutritional info per serving (15 radish pieces): Calories 85, Fat 6.7g, Net Carbs 3.6g, Protein 3.2g

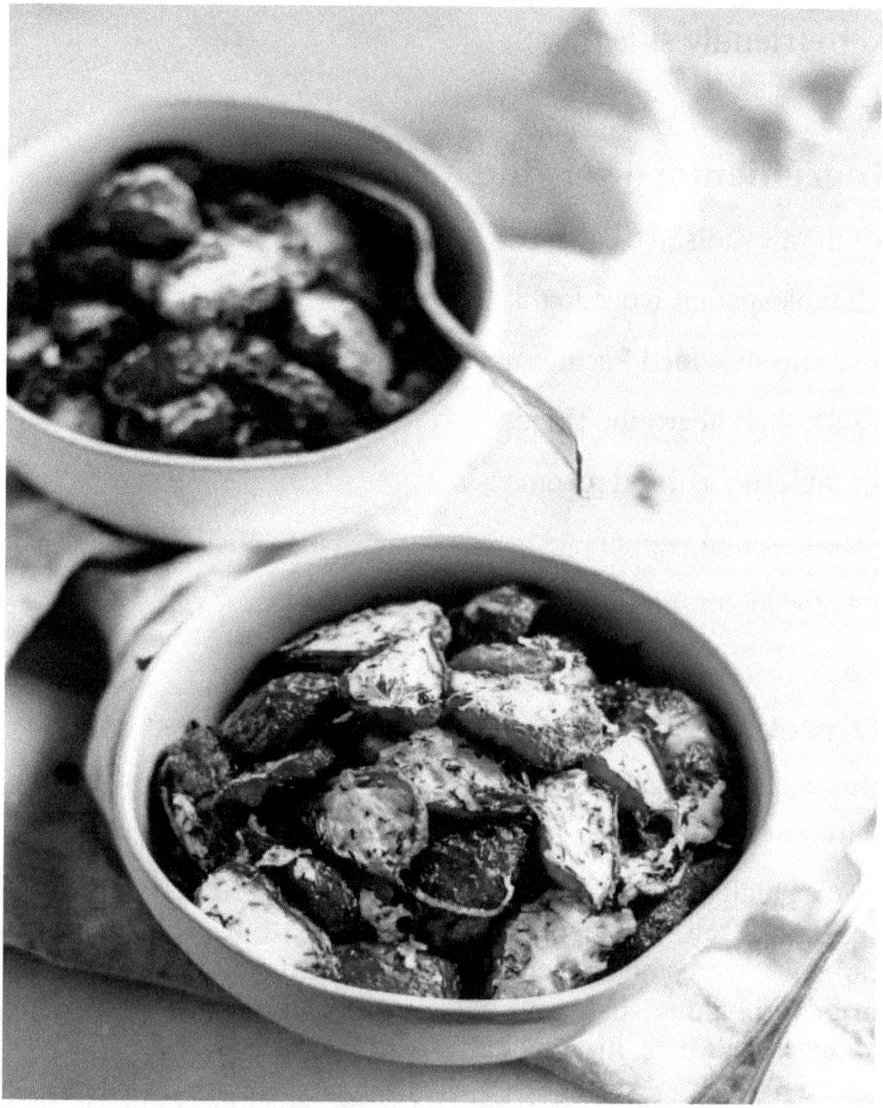

Desserts

Keto Vanilla Panna Cotta

Pure, unadulterated creaminess. For a luxurious keto dessert, look no further! Pomegranate and mint add holiday color, but you can enjoy this elegant, make-ahead finish to your celebrations year-round!

Ingredients: 4 servings

- 2 teaspoons unflavored powdered gelatin
- 2 cups heavy whipping cream
- 1 tablespoon vanilla extract
- 1 teaspoon erythritol
- 2 tablespoons pomegranate, the seeds
- Fresh mint
- Water

Directions:

• Soak the gelatin for 5-10 minutes in cold water. If you use powdered gelatin, mix it with cold water. Typically about 1 tablespoon water per teaspoon gelatin powder, but check the instructions for your specific brand. Set aside.

• Add cream, vanilla extract and erythritol to a saucepan and bring to a boil over medium heat. Lower the heat and let simmer for a couple of minutes on medium/low heat until the cream begins to thicken.

• Remove the cream from the heat and add the gelatin. If you're using sheets, be sure to squeeze as much water out of them as possible before adding to the cream. Stir until the gelatin has dissolved completely.

• Pour the cream into serving glasses. Allow to cool completely before covering with plastic wrap and placing in the fridge for 2 to 3 hours or overnight.

• Take the panna cotta out of the fridge half an hour before serving. Decorate with pomegranate seeds and fresh mint.

Nutritional info per serving: Calories 422, Fat 43g, Net Carbs 4g, Protein 4g

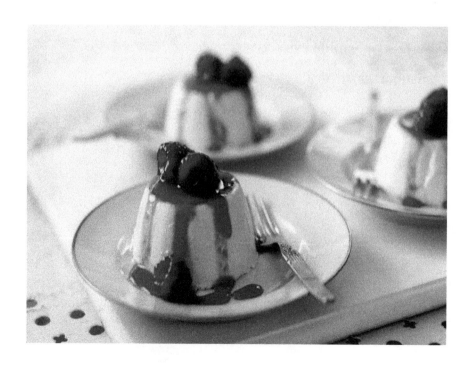

Almond Flour Keto Donuts

This low-carb donuts recipe with almond flour is super easy to make! These keto donuts taste just like regular sugar coated ones.

Ingredients: 6 donuts

Donuts:

• 1 cup almond flour

• 1 teaspoon cinnamon

• 1/3 cup erythritol

• ½ teaspoon vanilla extract

• ¼ cup butter, unsalted

• 2 large eggs

• 2 teaspoons gluten-free baking powder

• ¼ cup unsweetened almond milk

• 1/8 teaspoon sea salt

Cinnamon Coating:

• 1 teaspoon cinnamon

• 3 tablespoons butter, unsalted

• ½ cup erythritol

Directions:

• Preheat the oven to 350 degrees F. Grease a donut pan well.

• In a large bowl, stir together the almond flour, baking powder, erythritol, cinnamon and sea salt.

• In a small bowl, whisk together the melted butter, almond milk, eggs, and vanilla extract. Whisk the wet mixture into the dry mixture.

• Transfer the batter evenly into the donut cavities, filling them ¾ of the way. Bake for about 22-28 minutes, or longer for a silicone pan, until dark golden brown. Cool until donuts are easy to remove from the pan.

• Meanwhile, in a small bowl, stir together the erythritol and cinnamon for the coating.

• When the donuts have cooled enough to easily remove from the molds, transfer them to a cutting board. Brush both sides of one donut with butter, then press/roll in the sweetener/cinnamon mixture to coat. Repeat with the remaining donuts.

Nutritional info per serving: Calories 257, Fat 25g, Net Carbs 3g, Protein 6g

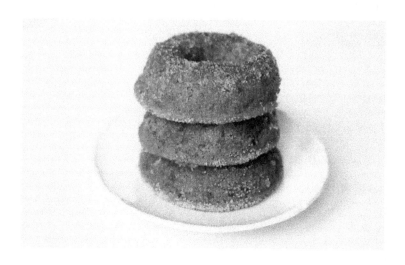

Cinnamon and Cardamom Fat Bombs

Small, but delicious! With familiar flavors of vanilla, cinnamon and cardamom, this is the perfect keto dessert!

Ingredients: 10 servings

- ¼ teaspoon ground cinnamon
- ¼ teaspoon ground cardamom
- ½ teaspoon vanilla extract
- 3 oz unsalted butter
- ½ cup unsweetened shredded coconut

Directions:

- Bring the butter to room temperature.
- Roast the shredded coconut carefully until they turn a little brown. This will create a delicious flavor, but you can skip this if you want. Let cool.
- Mix together butter, half of the shredded coconut and spices in a bowl.
- Form into walnut-sized balls with two teaspoons. Roll in the rest of the shredded coconut.
- Store in refrigerator or freezer.

Nutritional info per serving: Calories 90, Fat 10g, Net Carbs 0.4g, Protein 0.4g

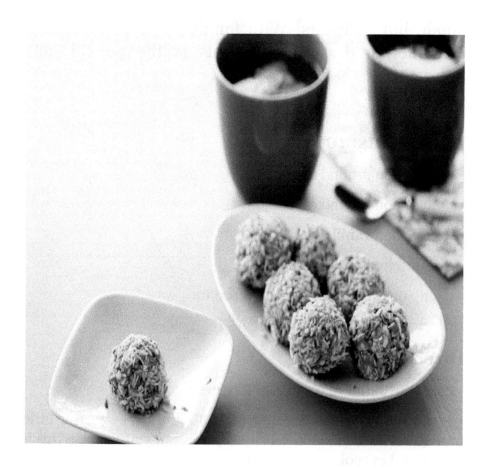

Keto Butter Pecan Cheesecake

This buttery rich keto pecan cheesecake is an attractive crowd-pleaser. Luscious pecan crust with a creamy and smooth cheesecake layer, perfect for festive occasions or whenever you need a new favorite desserts!

Ingredients: 4 servings

Cheesecake Crust:

- 1 tablespoon salted butter, melted

- 4 tablespoons pecans, finely crushed

- ½ tablespoon powdered erythritol

Filling:

- 4 tablespoons butter

- 4 tablespoons powdered erythritol

- 8 oz cream cheese, softened

- 1 egg, beaten

- 1 teaspoon vanilla extract

- 2 tablespoons unsweetened almond milk or heavy whipping cream

- Pecans, for garnishing

Directions:

• Preheat the oven to 350 degrees F.

• Grease a 4 inch springform pan with butter. Place melted butter, crushed pecans and confectioner's sweetener in a small bowl. Stir with a fork to combine well. Use your fingers to press mixture into the bottom of the springform pan.

• Place in the oven to pre-bake for 6 minutes while you prepare the filling.

• Place the butter in a small saucepan over medium/high heat. Stirring often, heat until the butter foams up and brown flecks appear. Remove from the heat and allow to cool a bit. This brown butter creates a caramel-like flavor to the cheesecake.

• Place softened cream cheese, confectioner's sweetener, almond milk or cream, egg and vanilla in a medium bowl. Use a hand mixer to combine well.

• Slowly add the browned butter and stir to combine. Pour mixture into pre-baked shell. Tent loosely with foil and bake for 30-35 minutes or until cheesecake is set and barely jiggles in the center.

• Remove from oven and allow to chill for 10 minutes then place in the fridge to chill for at least 2 hours.

• Store in an airtight container for up to 5 days.

Nutritional info per serving: Calories 383, Fat 39g, Net Carbs 4g, Protein 6g

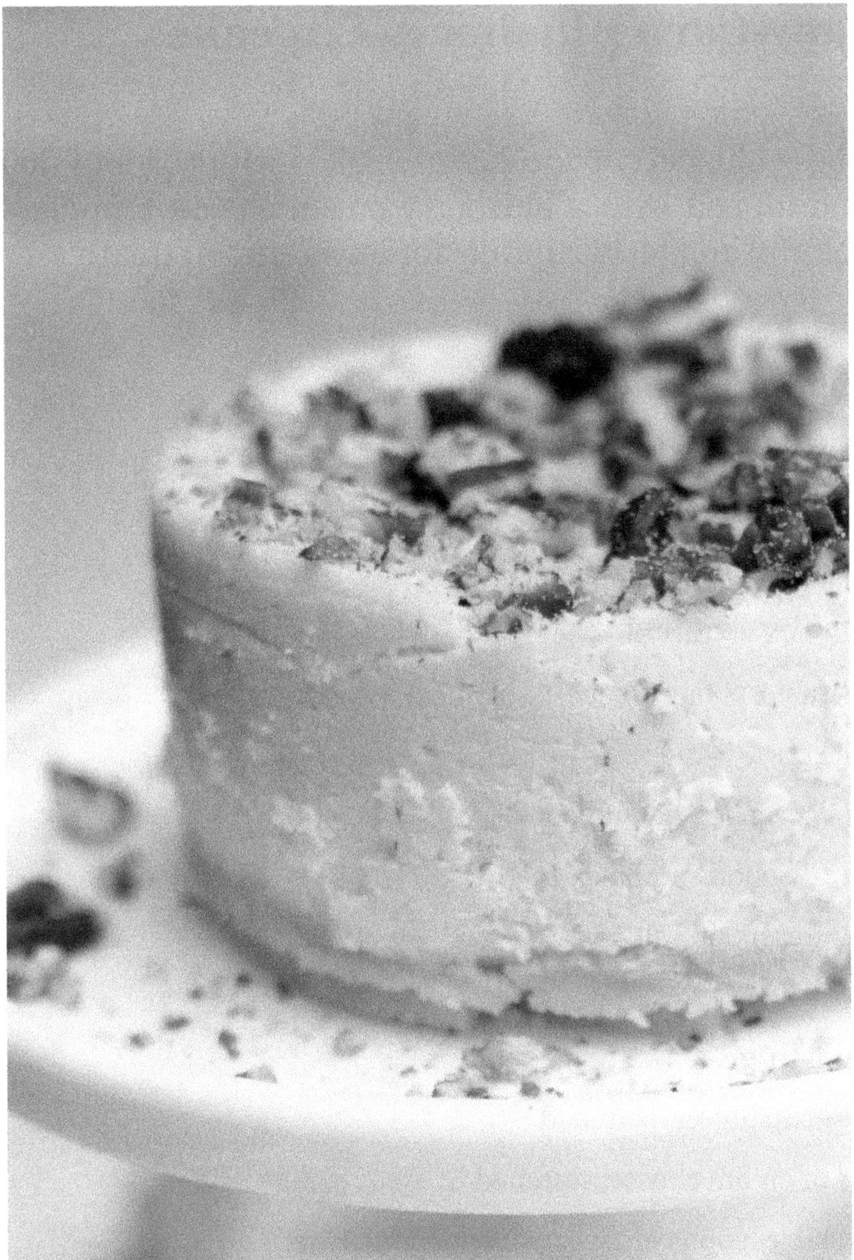

Low-Carb Blueberry Cupcakes

These blueberry cupcakes are baked with coconut flour and topped with a blueberry cream cheese topping. A colorful and tasty cupcake for an afternoon treat!

Ingredients: 6 cupcakes

Cupcake Mixture:

- ¼ cup butter, melted
- ¼ cup coconut flour
- ¼ cup erythritol
- 5 tablespoons blueberry blended mixture
- 3 eggs
- ½ teaspoon baking powder
- 1 teaspoon vanilla extract
- ¼ teaspoon salt

Frosting:

- ¼ cup butter, softened
- 4 oz cream cheese, softened
- 5 tablespoons blueberry blended mixture
- 1 tablespoon erythritol
- ½ teaspoon vanilla extract

Directions:

Blueberry Mixture:

• Place the blueberries in a blender and blitz. Set aside.

Cupcakes:

• Blend the butter, eggs, erythritol and vanilla essence.

• Add the coconut flour , baking powder and salt. Whisk until the batter is smooth.

• Add the blueberry mixture and combine thoroughly.

• Pour the batter into cupcake cups.

• Bake for 30 minutes until firm at 400 degrees F.

• Remove from the oven and allow to cool.

Frosting:

• Blend the butter, cream cheese, erythritol and vanilla until smooth.

• Add the blueberry blend and mix until combined. You might want to add more blueberries for a different color.

• Pipe or slather the mixture on top of the cupcakes. Eat and enjoy.

Nutritional info per serving (1 cupcake): Calories 253, Fat 23g, Net Carbs 4g, Protein 5g

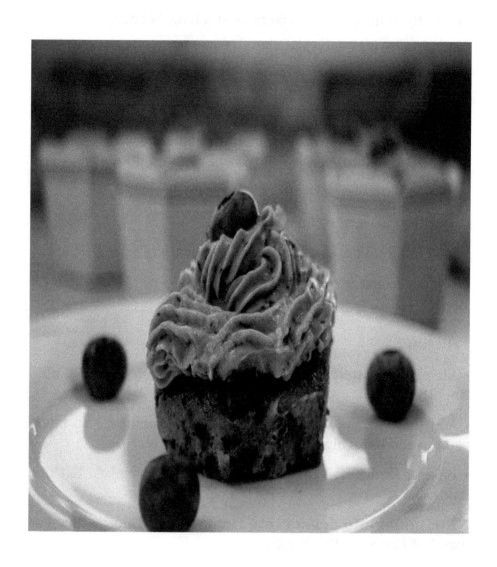

Keto Lemon Ice Cream

Treat the whole family to this fresh and creamy keto dessert. Summery homemade ice cream, bursting with luscious citrus flavor. Guaranteed sugar-free success!

Ingredients: 6 servings

- 1 lemon, zest and juice
- 1 ¾ cups heavy whipping cream
- 3 eggs
- 1/3 cup erythritol
- ¼ teaspoon yellow food coloring

Directions:

- Wash the lemon in lukewarm water. Finely grate the outer peel. Squeeze out the juice and set aside.

- Separate eggs. Beat egg whites until stiff. In another bowl, whisk egg yolks and sweetener until light and fluffy. Add lemon juice and a few drops of yellow food coloring. Carefully fold egg whites into yolk mixture.

- Whip cream in a large bowl until soft peaks form. Fold egg mixture into cream.

- Pour into ice cream maker and freeze according to manufacturer's instructions.

- If you don't have any ice cream maker, you can place the bowl in the freezer and give it a good stir every half hour until it reaches the desired consistency. It can take up to 2 hours. Use a spatula to scrape the inside of the bowl while stirring. If frozen, let stand at room temperature for 15 minutes before serving.

Nutritional info per serving: Calories 269, Fat 27g, Net Carbs 3g, Protein 5g

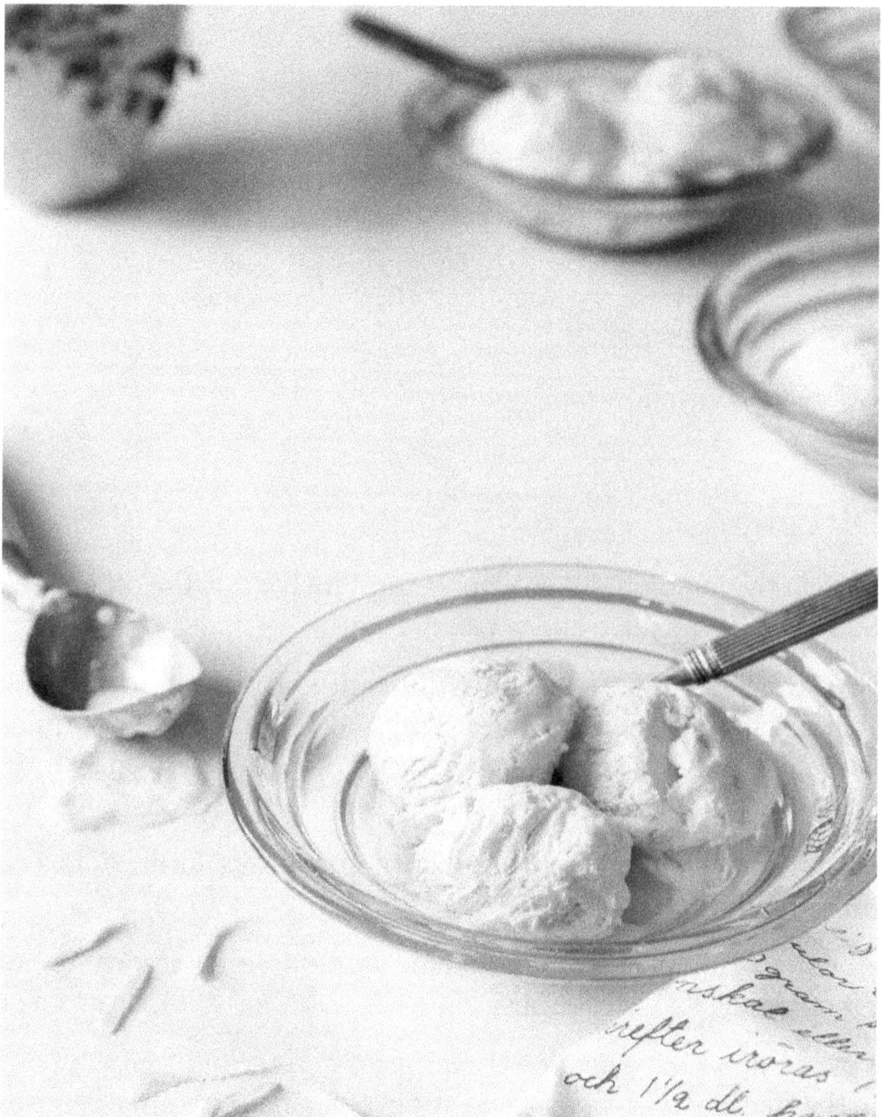

Sauces

Homemade Chicken Stock

Flavorful and comforting. Chicken stock is a hands-down stellar basic. Use it in sauces, stews, or soup for amazing flavor.

Ingredients: 4 servings

- 1 chicken
- 2 tablespoons olive oil
- 1 yellow onion
- 1 carrot
- 2 cloves garlic
- ½ cup white wine, dry
- 1 tablespoon dried thyme
- 1 teaspoon peppercorns, white
- 1 leek
- 1 bay leaf
- 6 cups water
- Salt

Directions:

• Peel and cut the vegetables into smaller pieces.

• Brown the vegetables in olive oil in a big pot, preferably one made of enamelled cast iron, until they have a nice color.

• Split the chicken down the middle and put both halves in the pot. Pour water and spices into the pot. Put the lid on, lower the heat, and let simmer for 2 hours.

• Take out the chicken and remove its bones. Save the meat.

• Spread out the chicken skin pieces on an oven sheet lined with parchment paper. Add spices to taste, and bake in the oven at 400 degrees F for about 15 minutes or until they are crispy.

• Crack the chicken bones and break up into smaller pieces. Put the bones back into the pot and simmer for about 3 more hours.

• Filter the stock through a fine strainer and pour the stock back into the pot. Reduce to half or more, depending on how rich you want your stock to be. The stock isn't supposed to boil vigorously. Just let it simmer over medium/low heat. Season with salt to taste towards the end.

• Store in the fridge for 2-3 days or freeze in a smaller packages for up to 3 months. It's perfect to use as a natural flavor enhancer in soups, pots and sauces.

Using the Slow Cooker:

If you have a slow cooker, it is wonderful for making stock. Leave the chicken in one piece and combine the ingredients in a slow cooker. Cook on high for 3 hours. Remove the meat, switch temperature to low, and cook the bones for at least 8 more hours (the longer, the better). Add to a saucepan without a lid and reduce on low to medium heat until you reach the desired concentration.

Nutritional info per serving: Calories 145, Fat 13g, Net Carbs 0.5g, Protein 7g

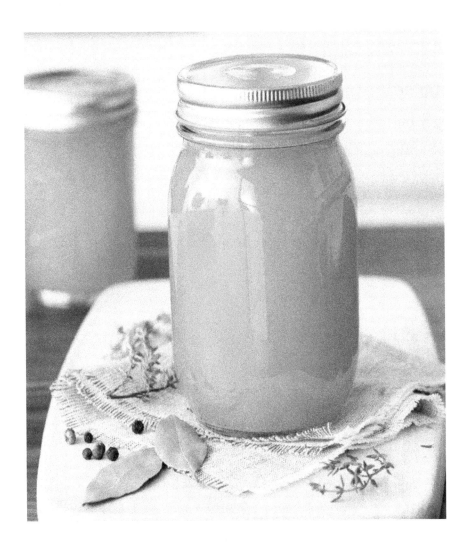

Herb Butter

Fresh herbs. Lemony butter. Try this keto classic spread on anything from meat to fish to veggies!

Ingredients: 4 servings

• 5 oz butter, at room temperature

• ½ tablespoon garlic powder

• 1 clove garlic, pressed

• 4 tablespoons fresh parsley, finely chopped

• 1 teaspoon lemon juice

• ½ teaspoon salt

Directions:

• Mix all ingredients thoroughly in a small bowl. Set aside for 15 minutes to let the flavors develop before serving. If you prepare this ahead of time you should store it in the refrigerator.

Nutritional info per serving: Calories 258, Fat 28g, Net Carbs 1g, Protein 1g

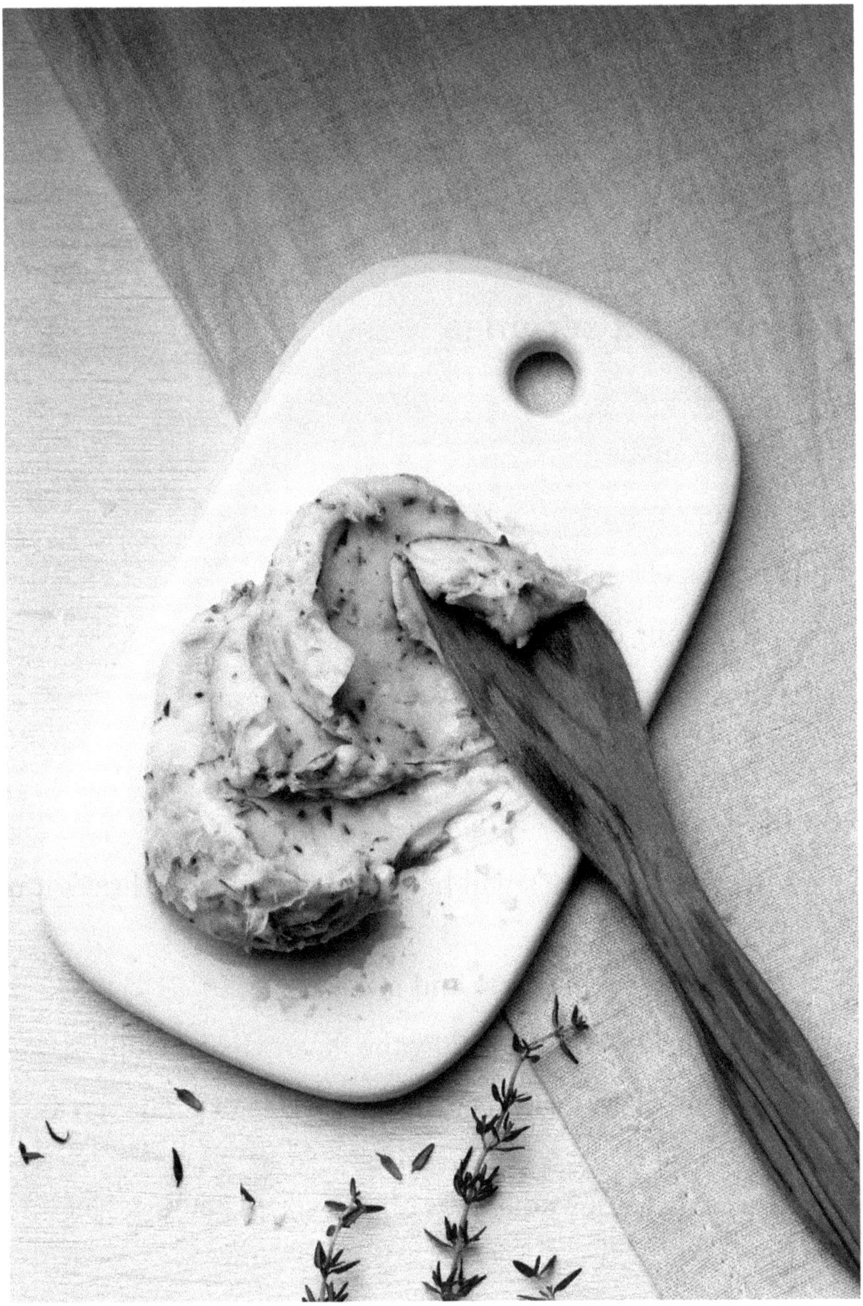

Keto Blue Cheese Dressing

Wonderfully creamy and so versatile! Enjoy this tangy keto sauce on salads, meat, or chicken. And it works as a super tasty dip for veggies.

Ingredients: 4 servings

• 5 oz blue cheese

• ½ cup mayonnaise

• ¾ cup Greek yogurt

• 2 tablespoons fresh parsley, finely chopped

• Heavy whipping cream or water

• Salt and pepper to taste

Directions:

• Place the cheese into a small bowl and use a fork to break it up into coarse chunks.

• Add yogurt and mayonnaise and mix well.

• Let sit for a few minutes to allow the flavors to develop.

• Salt and pepper to taste. Dilute with water or heavy cream if needed.

Nutritional info per serving: Calories 375, Fat 36g, Net Carbs 3g, Protein 9g

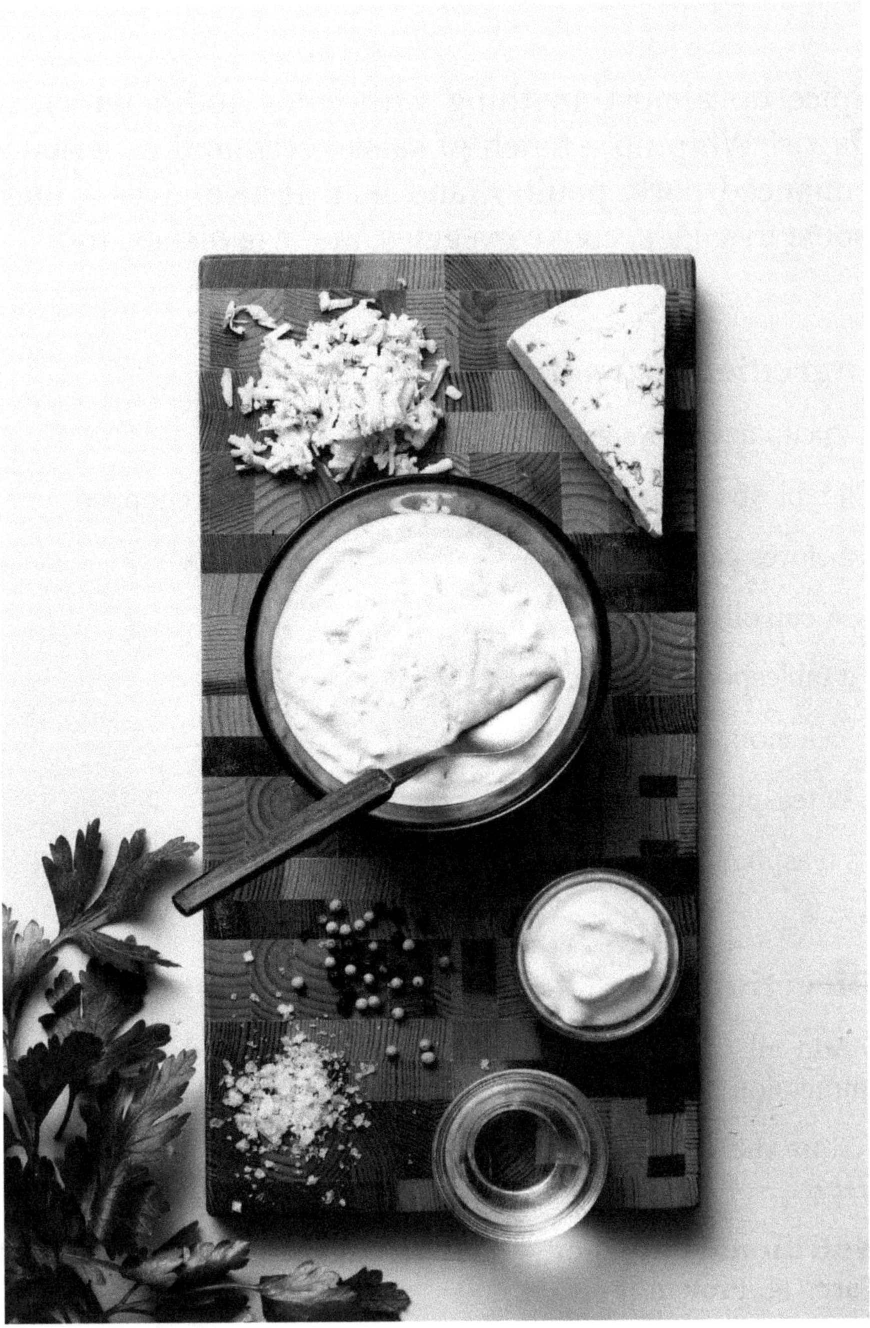

Keto Salsa Verde

Spice up almost anything with color and a punch of flavor! Whip up a batch of salsa verde and experience enhanced pork, poultry, and fish. It also gives a huge boost to salads, cooked veggies, and egg dishes, too!

Ingredients: 4 servings

- ½ cup fresh parsley, finely chopped
- 3 tablespoons fresh basil or fresh cilantro, finely chopped
- 2 cloves garlic, crushed
- ¾ cup olive oil
- 2 tablespoons small capers
- ½ lemon, the juice
- ½ teaspoon ground black pepper
- 1 teaspoon sea salt

Directions:

- Add all of the ingredients to a deep bowl and mix with an immersion blender until the sauce has the desired consistency.

- Store the sauce in the refrigerator for up to 4-5 days or in the freezer.

Nutritional info per serving: Calories 363, Fat 40g, Net Carbs 1g, Protein 1g

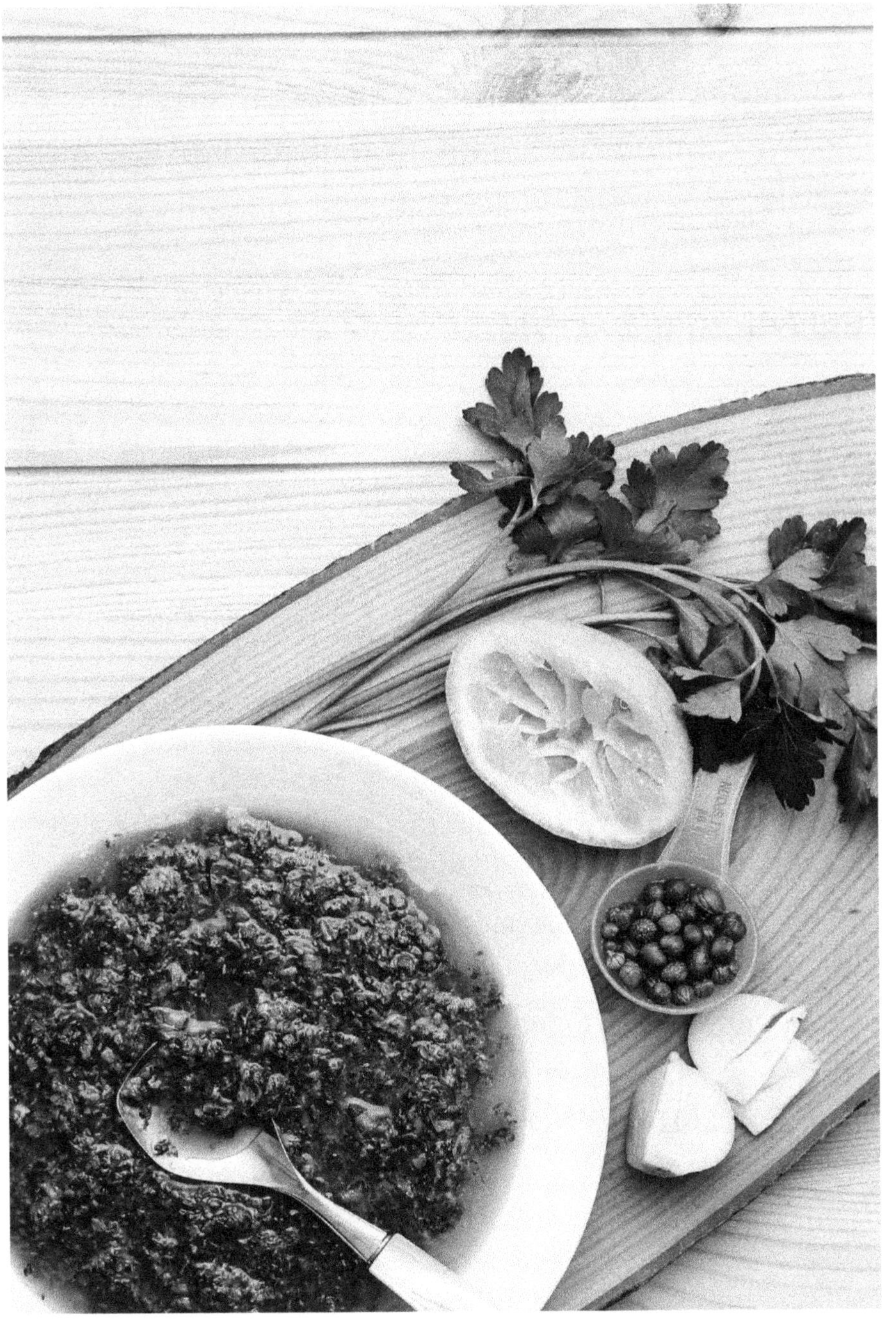

Parmesan Butter

This simple keto combination is equal parts salty and creamy. Fabulous with both meat dishes and vegetarian meals!

Ingredients: 4 servings

- 5 1/3 oz butter
- 2 oz grated Parmesan cheese
- ¼ teaspoon ground black pepper
- ½ teaspoon salt

Directions:

• Let the butter reach room temperature.

• Mix all ingredients with a fork in a small bowl. Set aside for 15 minutes to allow the flavors to develop.

• Serve the butter as a condiment and let it melt over meat, chicken, fish or vegetables.

• The butter will keep for at least one week and may also be stored in the freezer.

Nutritional info per serving: Calories 328, Fat 34g, Net Carbs 1g, Protein 6g

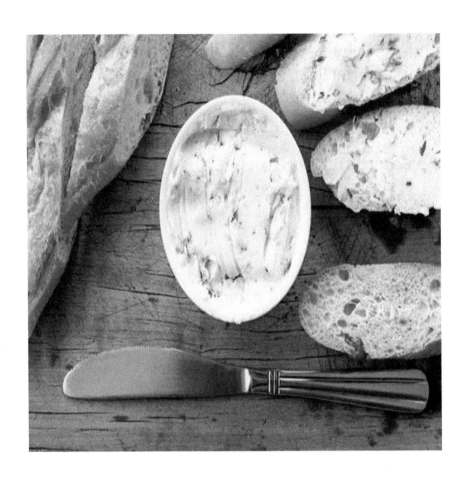

Low-Carb Guacamole

A little guacamole just makes life better! This foolproof recipe is perfect for a snack with veggies or on top of grilled chicken or burgers.

Ingredients: 4 servings

- 2 ripe avocados
- 1 clove garlic
- 3 tablespoons olive oil
- ½ white onion
- 1 tomato, diced
- 5 1/3 tablespoons fresh cilantro
- ½ lime, the juice
- Salt and pepper

Directions:

• Peel the avocados and mash with a fork. Grate or chop the onion finely and add to the mash. Squeeze the lime and add the juice.

• Add tomato, olive oil and finely chopped cilantro. Season with salt and pepper and mix well.

Nutritional info per serving: Calories 264, Fat 25g, Net Carbs 5g, Protein 3g

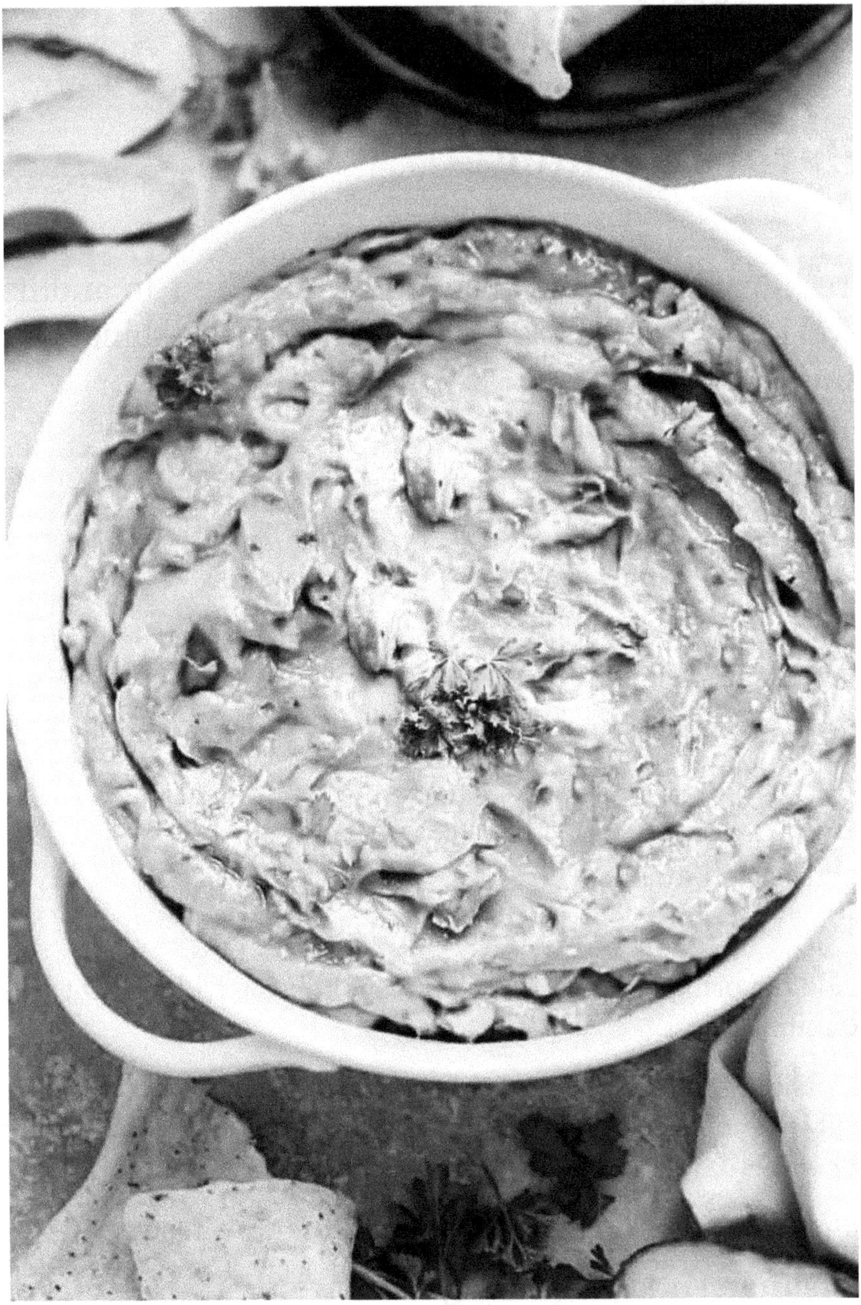

Drinks

Flavored Water

Fresh, cold water! Try elevating your water to another level by adding fruit, berries or herbs! Refreshing, tasty and close to 0 carbs!

Ingredients: 4 servings

• 4 cups cold water

• flavoring of your choice, for example fresh raspberries or fresh mint or sliced cucumber

• 2 cups ice cubes

Directions:

• Pour fresh, cold water into a pitcher.

• Add flavoring of your choice and let sit in the fridge for at least 30 minutes.

• Possible additions include berries, fruit, fresh mint, or citrus fruit like orange, grapefruit, lime and lemon in thin slices. Cucumber is another classic with a neutral but refreshing taste.

• Just a few slices or pieces will flavor an entire pitcher.

Nutritional info per serving: Calories 0, Fat 0g, Net Carbs 0g, Protein 0g

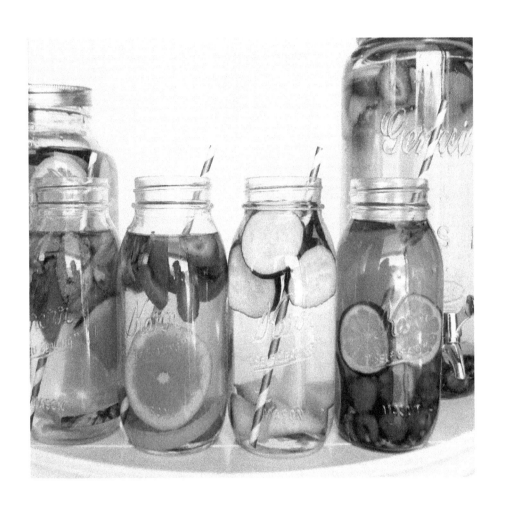

Chamomile Mint Tea

This tea is delicious by itself, and it also has some health benefits. Chamomile soothes stomach pains and helps you to get to sleep. And peppermint is great for digestive troubles.

Ingredients: 1 serving

• 1 teaspoon chamomile flowers

• 1 teaspoon peppermint leaves

• 1 cup boiling water

Directions:

• Add the chamomile and peppermint to a tea pot or mug and pour in the boiling water.

• Infuse for 4-5 minutes, remove the herbs and drink.

Nutritional info per serving: Calories 0, Fat 0g, Net Carbs 0g, Protein 0g

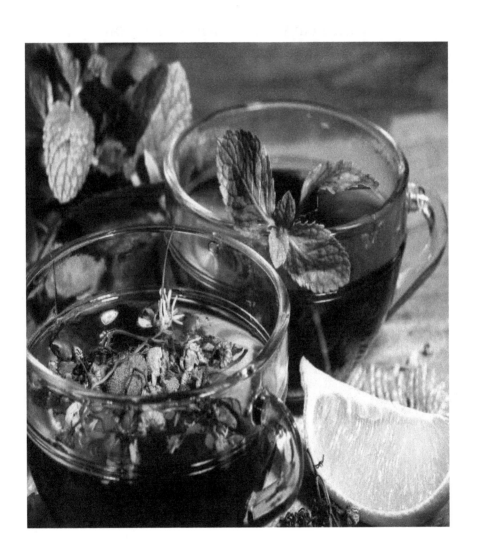

Coffee with Cream

Hot coffee with heavy cream will warm you up to your toes! Try this in the morning, as a mid-day boost, or as a decadent and creamy keto dessert!

Ingredients: 4 servings

• 3 cups coffee, brewed the way you like it

• 1 cup heavy whipping cream

Directions:

• Make your coffee the way you like it. Pour the cream in a small saucepan and heat gently while stirring until it's frothy.

• Pour the warm cream in a big cup, add coffee and stir. Serve straight away as is, or with a handful of nuts or a piece of cheese.

Nutritional info per serving: Calories 206, Fat 22g, Net Carbs 2g, Protein 2g

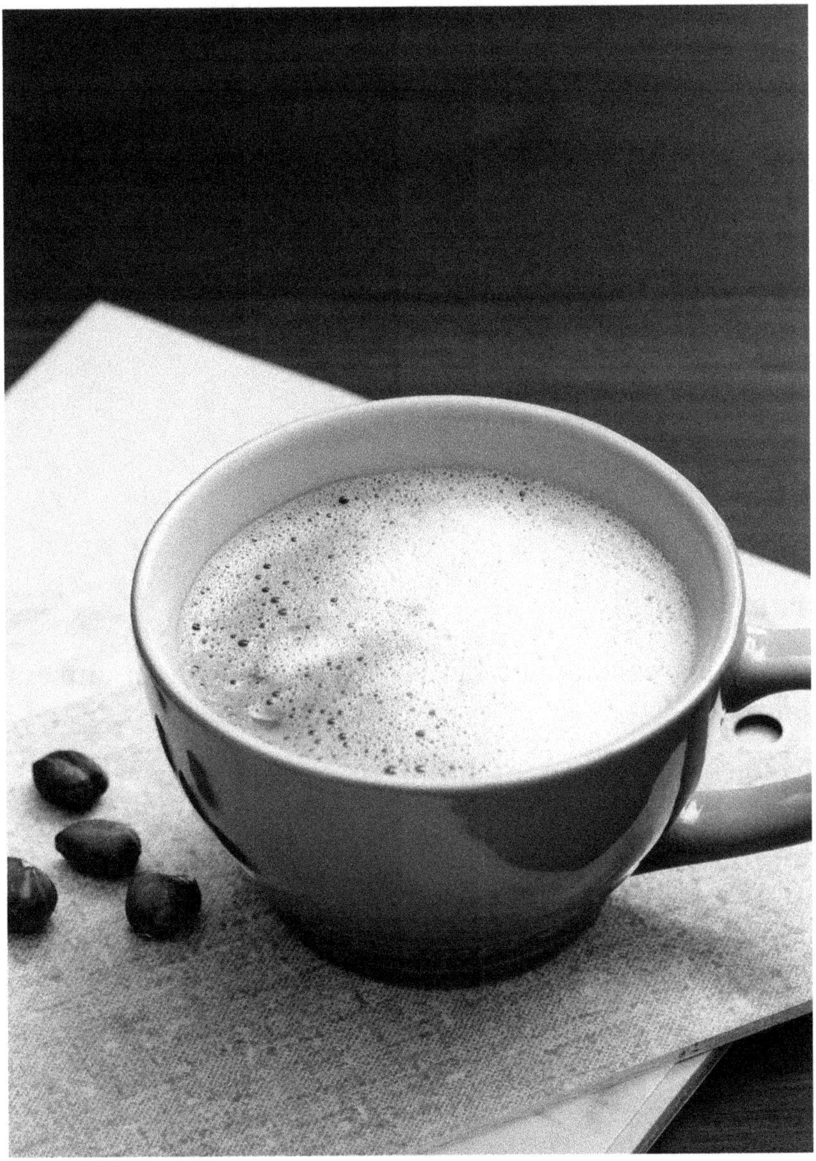

Keto Hot Chocolate

Insane chocolate creaminess in a cup! Pure keto love!

Ingredients: 1 serving

- 1 tablespoon cocoa powder
- 1 oz unsalted butter
- ¼ teaspoon vanilla extract
- 1 teaspoon powdered erythritol
- 1 cup boiling water

Directions:

• Put the ingredients in a tall beaker to use with an immersion blender.

• Mix for 15-20 seconds or until there's a fine foam on top.

• Pour the hot cocoa carefully into cups and enjoy.

Nutritional info per serving: Calories 216, Fat 23g, Net Carbs 1g, Protein 1g

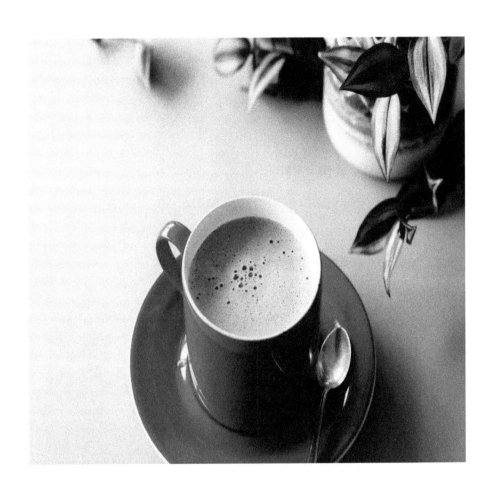

Vanilla Caramel Frappuccino

Vanilla caramel frappuccino is a super frosty, treat beverage. This is a versatile recipe that is simple to make in the blender.

Ingredients: 2 servings

- 1 cup coffee, cool or at room temperature
- 2 cups unsweetened almond milk or coconut milk
- ¼ teaspoon vanilla extract
- 4 teaspoons sweetener of your choice
- 4 tablespoons heavy whipping cream
- 3 cups ice

Caramel Sauce:

- 1 tablespoon sweetener of your choice
- 2 tablespoons heavy cream
- 2 tablespoons butter
- ¼ teaspoon molasses

Directions:

- In a small saucepan on medium heat, add all the caramel sauce ingredients and melt and stir to combine. Turn up to medium/high heat and stir until it starts to bubble and thicken. Remove from heat to cool. Set aside.

• In a blender add coffee, almond milk or coconut milk, vanilla extract, 2 to 3 teaspoons sweetener of choice, and half of the caramel sauce. Blend until mixed.

• Add ice to the blender and blend until smooth.

• Pour into a glass, top with whipped cream and drizzle with remainder of reserved caramel sauce.

Nutritional info per serving: Calories 300, Fat 29g, Net Carbs 6g, Protein 4g

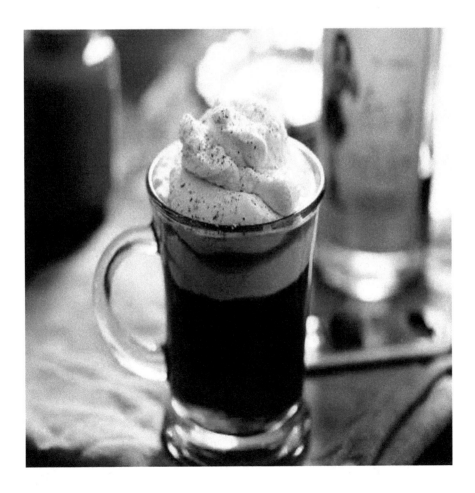

CPSIA information can be obtained
at www.ICGtesting.com
Printed in the USA
BVHW091056220221
600778BV00007B/745

9 781914 371257